THE ILLNESS IS THE CURE

Maya Christobel
720-421-5004

THE ILLNESS IS THE CURE

an introduction to

LIFE MEDICINE &

LIFE DOCTORING

a new existential approach to illness

Peter Wilberg

ISBN-13: 978-1466417540

ISBN-10: 1466417544

Disclaimer

This radical critique of biological medicine is in no way intended to invalidate the good intent and caring efforts of countless physicians, nurses and other health professionals operating within institutions dominated by the biomedical belief system. Its only aim is to help release them – and their patients – from the iron grip of that system. Nor, despite the scepticism of health professional towards any type of 'psychological' approach to medicine, does this book seek to deny that for those who continue to have trust in biological treatments – and/or suffer less from side effects from them than most – such treatments can themselves serve as a form of temporary quick-fix psychological medicine i.e. a 'placebo'.

CONTENTS

PART 1
INTRODUCTION

Questions for the Reader

Have you ever felt that by simply making an appointment to see your doctor you are just bothering them and interfering with their busy schedule?

Have you ever felt your doctor's sole purpose in listening to you is to come to the quickest possible way of seeing you out – whether by handing out a prescription or arranging a test?

Have you ever felt frustrated by the lack of truly patient listening time that doctors are able or willing to give you?

Have you ever felt infantilised or treated like a child by medical professionals?

Have you ever felt that there was no time for your questions to be fully heard or answered?

 Have you ever felt confused by often dramatically conflicting opinions and beliefs expressed by different doctors and consultants?

Have you ever felt frustrated about being given one medical test after another, being passed from one anonymous consultant to another, or being given one form of treatment or surgery after another – all without ever having a say in what is going on?

Have you ever felt that your direct felt experience of your illness was of no interest to medical professionals or 'experts'?

Have you ever felt so scared by a medical diagnosis such as cancer that it has made you feel ill – even though you might have been feeling fine or even had absolutely no symptoms at all beforehand?

Have you ever suffered acute or chronic side effects from medical drugs and treatments that you were not warned about - or that were largely ignored?

Have you ever wondered at the high cost of health insurance, drugs and treatments – and why it is that even publicly funded health institutions and services are constantly in financial crisis?

Has it ever occurred to you that illness is a source of huge profits for drug companies, the corporate health industry as a whole, and even promoters of health 'supplements' or 'alternative' medicine?

Have you ever considered that illness itself may at least partly be an expression of life as people are economically pressured to live it in a fundamentally sick and money-driven society?

Have you ever suspected that the timing and nature of your illness was not accidental but had to do with events that had been going on in your life and feelings associated with them?

Have you ever felt, as a medical practitioner, that there may be a lot more to a patient's symptoms or illness than meets the medical eye - but that your training has not equipped you to explore it, and that your job and institutional environment give you no time or encouragement to do so?

If so, then read on....

Guiding Thoughts

"An advanced industrial society is sick-making because it disables people from coping with their environment and, when they break down, it substitutes a 'clinical' prosthesis for the broken relationships."

"People would rebel against such an environment if medicine did not explain their biological disorientation as a defect in their health, rather than as a defect in the way of life which is imposed on them or which they impose on themselves."

"A number of authors have ... tried to debunk the status of mental deviance as a 'disease'. Paradoxically, they have rendered it more and not less difficult to raise the same kind of question about <u>disease in general</u>."

Ivan Illich

"The idea of one basis for Science and another for Life is from the very outset a lie."

Karl Marx

"There is not much difference whether a human being is looked on as a 'case' or as a number to be tattooed on the arm."

from *Doctors of Infamy - on the perversion of medicine in the Third Reich*

"Patients turn their problems into illnesses, and ... the physician's job is to turn them back into problems."

Michael Balint

"...the body's symptoms are not necessarily pathological, that is, they are not just sicknesses which must be healed, repressed or cured. Symptoms are potentially meaningful and purposeful conditions... as well as a royal road into the development of the personality."

Arnold Mindell

"A psychological medicine ... obviously comes into conflict with the technological development of medicine, which has already become an Über-technology. This development is itself closely connected with modern economic structures, with industry, with the income sources of physicians, with the gigantic need for patients – and others – to be deceived."

"That illnesses have meaning, can lead those affected to the meaning of their lives – this is the insight that natural-scientific medicine has fundamentally impeded."

"One sees, now, that psychology in medicine brings forth an unexpected result. It does not only bring knowledge of the soul, but illuminates the body in such a way as to let it appear in a new light. The body is no longer what it seemed before, and what anatomy and physiology teach."

"Illness can be experienced as this – that through a bodily occurrence a development in awareness is created."

"The greatest goal would be to understand how in every case, in what way an illness is just a muted final thought, a still insufficiently [fulfilled] creative act."

Viktor von Weizsäcker

"... the genetic approach is clear to everyone. It seems self-evident. But it suffers from a deficit, which is all too easily and therefore all too often overlooked. To be in a position to explain an illness genetically, we need first of all to explain what the illness in itself _is_."

"Those who wish to stick rigidly to genetic explanation, without first of all clarifying the essence of that which they wish to explain, can be compared to people who wish to reach a goal, without first of all bringing this goal in view."

"It can be that a true understanding of the essence of an illness...prohibits all causal-genetic explanation...."

"It is of the highest importance that there be thinking physicians, who are not of a mind to leave the field for the scientific technologists."

Martin Heidegger

"If people become ill, it is quite fashionable to say that the immunity system has temporarily failed – yet the body itself knows that certain 'dis-eases' are healthy reactions. The body does not recognise <u>diseases as diseases</u> in usually understood terms."

"You are not healthy ... no matter how robust your physical condition, if your relationships are unhealthy, unsatisfying, frustrating or hard to achieve."

"...try to understand that the particular dilemma of illness is not an event forced upon you ... Rather realise that to some extent or another your dilemma or your illness <u>has been chosen by you</u>...

"There is no need to feel guilty since you <u>meant very well</u> as you made each choice..."

"... no person dies ahead of his or her time. The individual chooses the time of death."

"...no individual dies of cancer or AIDS, or any other condition, until they themselves have set the time."

from *The Way Toward Health* – a Seth book by Jane Roberts

The Basic Questions

- What if 'explaining' an illness is one thing, but *understanding* it is quite another?
- What if illnesses have *life meanings* and not just scientific 'explanations' and biological 'causes'?
- What if the *biology* of the human body cannot be separated from the *biography* of the human being?
- What if *the life of the human body* cannot in any way be separated from *the life of the human being* in all its existential dimensions – personal, social and economic?
- What if *body symptoms* are like *dream symbols* – there to be understood and to tell us something?
- **What if 'the illness is the cure'** – offering patients an opportunity to gain important insights into themselves to bring about healing transformations in their *lives* and not just their bodies?
- What if conventional biomedical tests and treatments aimed at finding ways to fight and 'cure' a person's illness can prevent them from learning vital lessons from their illness?
- What if official medical statistics show that conventional forms of biomedical treatment are themselves a leading cause of death?
- What if many prescription drugs worsen or prolong the very symptoms they are prescribed for?
- What if so-called 'scientific' medicine is really *money-driven medicine* – relying on illness as a cash cow for the corporate health industry?

- What if every *bodily state* is at the same time a *state of consciousness* – and vice versa – thus making nonsense of the separation between 'body' and 'mind', medical treatments on the one hand and psychological therapies on the other?

Then we would need a new understanding of illness and a new model of medicine – one that not only questions but goes beyond the biomedical model.

- This in turn could spare both individuals and private and public health services the huge costs of pharmaceutical drugs and hi-tech biomedical equipment.
- It would also mean that psychological counsellors and therapists could no longer leave 'medical' problems and symptoms to the medical profession.
- Indeed it would allow a new foundation for *medical training* to be created – not biological medicine but 'Life Medicine'.
- Out of this could come very different ways of treating patients – not through conventional doctoring but through 'Life Doctoring'. For the aim of Life Medicine and the Life Doctor is to help patients discover in what ways their *illness is the cure* – there to help them *heal their lives.*
- In this way the individual patient would no longer be reduced to 'a case' of some generic 'disease'. Instead every such 'case' and every such 'disease' would be understood in terms of the individual life circumstances behind it.

Medicine, Life and Science

In a way intended to be of help to both patients and health professionals, this book challenges one of the most basic assumptions shared by almost *all* forms of medicine – conventional or 'alternative', 'scientific', 'traditional' or 'spiritual'. This is the assumption that illness is something to *be cured* rather than *being the cure*.

To challenge this basic assumption, I introduce a fundamentally new 'existential' approach to health and illness which I call 'Life Medicine' and 'Life Doctoring'. Life Doctoring and Life Medicine offer patients opportunities to come to an understanding of how and in what ways their *illness is itself the cure* – offering a source of new *healing understandings* of themselves and a *healing transformation* of their lives.

For in contrast to both 'orthodox' and 'alternative' medicine – each of which in their own ways seek nothing but 'causes' and 'cures' for illness – Life Medicine and Life Doctoring do not *separate* science and life, biology from biography, the life of the *human body* and the life of the *human being.* Instead the focus is on the larger *life context* and *specific life meanings* that particular symptoms and illnesses hold for the individual patient. For as Marx wrote:

"The idea of one basis for science and another for life is from the very outset a lie."

This 'lie' unfortunately has dire consequences of which too few are aware. For research by the medical establishment itself has shown that conventional biomedical diagnosis and treatment through drugs and surgery is itself *the* leading cause of premature death – ahead of both cancer and heart disease.

By offering an entirely new framework for understanding health and illness, Life Medicine and Life Doctoring can help patients to not only understand the underlying sense of 'dis-ease' in their *lives* that lies behind their illness. Life Medicine and Life Doctoring can also serve a vital *preventative* role by (a) preventing this 'dis-ease' manifesting further as clinical 'disease', and (b) educating patients about the possible dangers and potentially sickness-causing or 'iatrogenic' effects of many standard forms of biomedical testing and treatment.

Both biomedical and 'alternative' explanations of illness are comparable in many respects to the way in which scientists sought to 'explain' dreams before Freud – denying them all *meaning*. Yet what if the symptoms are comparable to disturbing dream symbols and experiences – both expressions of a felt 'dis-ease'? What if illnesses are a type of embodied dream or 'body dream'? Then deep *understanding* and not just medical-scientific 'explanation', testing and treatment is required.

For again, to 'explain' an illness is one thing. Yet to *understand* it is quite another. For understanding has to do with *meaning*. Yet so-called 'biological' medicine does not even recognise or understand the root meaning of the very term 'biology' itself – which does not refer to a set of specialist sciences, but rather to the 'speech' (Greek *logos*) of 'life' (Greek *bios*). Speech carries and communicates meaning. Nothing could be further from the root meaning of 'biology' then, than the so-called biological 'sciences' – which reduce the life, language and 'speech' of the human body itself to a mere molecular 'expression' of its genes.

That is why, as Martin Heidegger wrote: *"The essential realm in which biology moves can never be grounded in biology as a science."* For the realm in which biology moves is a realm of living and embodied meaning. In contrast, what most fundamentally defines the 'biomedical model' of medicine – based as it is on "biology as a science" – is the way it totally denies any *personal life meaning* to illness – and in particular the exact timing, life situation and larger life context in which an individual's symptoms first emerge. On the contrary, by merely seeking to fit a person's symptoms into the frame of wholly impersonal diagnostic or statistical criteria, and then treating their illness with no less impersonal methods of drug or hi-tech treatment, biomedicine can *aggravate* the very sense of *personal meaning loss* that lies behind most illnesses – as well as damaging rather than healing patients' bodies, and even endangering their lives.

The continuing *monopoly* of biomedicine over our entire understanding of and approach to illness has one reason and one reason only – namely that it is not actually 'science driven' but 'money driven' – turning illness into a source of vast profits for the drug companies and manufacturers of hi-tech medical equipment. Indeed 'health' itself is increasingly defined merely in monetary terms – as the patient's capacity for 'employment' as a wage-slave and to 'function' economically as a profit-source for employers.

Many people are concerned about the rising costs of public health care or angered by a global trend towards the privatisation of health services. Yet the roots of this trend lie in the fact that *illness itself* has long been 'privatised' – seen as bearing no relation at all to the social and economic 'ills' affecting the patient. To declare that 'the illness is the cure' is also to recognise that the 'cause' of illness does not lie in the individual alone but also in the world – and that illness itself is in part a *healthy* response to a fundamentally *sick world* – and this way also helps to *heal* that world.

PART 2
ON BIOLOGICAL MEDICINE

Medicine and Meaning

"Modern medical science largely considers the human body to be a kind of mechanical model, a sort of vehicle like a car that needs to be checked by a garage every so often."

from *The Way Toward Health* by Jane Roberts

A driver who for some reason is in a hurry to get somewhere decides to 'run the red light' at a junction, and has an accident. Yet would we even think of seeking to explain their consequent injuries purely as a result of automobile mechanics, for example suspecting the possibility of 'faulty pedals' or some other mechanical defect – seeing this as what 'caused' the car to go through the red light (and then subjecting the car to a whole series of diagnostic tests).* This would seem absurd to common sense - and yet it is no less absurd than seeing the body as a mechanical vehicle – like a car – and treating illness as something caused by a technical fault in some part of that vehicle.

For cars also have drivers. To be sure, the driver in our example made a choice, whereas we do not normally think of ourselves as 'choosing' to get ill. Yet the driver's choice itself was no doubt a response to a current or overall *life situation*. The driver might have been in a hurry for some reason, for example late for work or for a job interview. The decision to run the red light may not even have been a fully conscious or premeditated decision – simply a more or less aware bodily reaction to the specific life situation itself. Nevertheless shooting the red light was a choice.

What if the same applies to illness? Namely that there is a way in which we do not so much consciously 'choose' as subconsciously 'accede' to getting ill, albeit in a particular life context and for particular life reasons that are quite conscious to us: for example a pressing need to get a job – or even a subconscious desire to use the illness as a way of taking 'time out' from the pressures of life and/or receiving care and attention. Whatever the possible *meaning* of the accident/illness might be for a specific individual there is one thing we can be sure of however – there *is* such a meaning – and that just seeking, however thoroughly, for a mechanical fault in the individual's bodily 'vehicle' *will never reveal it.*

Indeed even *were* such a mechanical fault to be discovered or diagnosed, it might itself be the result of a subconscious decision on the part of our 'driver' in response to a situation arising in their life journey i.e. something that in some way *drove* them to neglect that vehicle or ignore its warning signs. Simply taking the vehicle to a garage and repairing the fault will therefore not address its true meaning or that of its possible consequences. For these have to do with the life circumstances of the human being and not the mechanics or 'biology' of his bodily vehicle alone. Simply to say, for example, that the driver got a dodgy vehicle with an inherited 'fault', that they neglected it or abused it through mishandling – or that they failed to put it through a regular medical 'MOT' – is not enough. For the question 'why?' still remains – a question of life motive and meaning and not a mere matter of some inherited biological or mechanical 'defect', 'accident', or sequence of 'cause and effect'.

Even for our hypothetical driver who ends up in hospital due to a serious 'accident' the result might be a highly meaningful and life-changing one in a positive sense, allowing him or her to *re-think their life* and not just receive treatment for their body. Yet this simple but basic distinction – between the life of the human being and its expression in the life of the human body – is consistently ignored by medical science and biological medicine – which by seeking explanations for illness purely in terms of defects of our bodily 'vehicle' blocks all forms of research into the *meaning* of illness. For even if a defect is found in the form of some medically recognised 'disease' or 'disorder', biological medicine cannot yet explain the cause of the disease or disorder itself – except in terms of some genetic defect. Yet not even any form of genetic explanation can actually explain why one *individual and not another* should contract a particular disease. For just as not everyone who smokes gets lung cancer, and not everyone falls ill from an epidemic, neither does everyone with an errant gene end up with the disease associated with it.

*acknowledgement to Andrew Gara for this significant analogy

What Biological Medicine Can't Explain

The more biological medicine seeks to 'scientifically' explain illness – the more it leaves *unexplained.*

Examples:

Why one individual and not another contracts a particular disease – even though they may share the same genes thought to be its 'cause' or the same 'unhealthy' habits such as smoking.

Why some people never get 'infected' by others, even those living closest to them or even in the midst of widespread epidemics or pandemics.

Why biomedical treatment is itself *a leading cause of death* ahead of cancer, stroke and heart disease.

Why 'successful' drug treatment or surgery for illness often precipitates mental psychosis or precedes the emergence of new symptoms just as serious as the original ones.

Why the greatest danger period for mental and physical health patients occurs after finishing a 'successful' course of medical treatment and being told that they are well.

Why social isolation is a greater risk factor for health and lowers life expectancy more than smoking, diet or obesity.

Why support groups for women with breast cancer patients have been found to double their life expectancy.

Why support from a spouse dramatically improves survival rates from heart transplants.

Why so many illnesses occur after or often on the exact anniversary of significant life events – such as bereavements, the end of a relationship, the start or loss of a job, taking an exam, retirement or even just going on holiday.

Why there is an 80% correlation between stressful life events and the onset of an illness in the two years following those events.

Why the chances of simply getting a cold are increased by life difficulties or disappointments, in particular those to do with employment or relationship problems.

Why the incidence of previously widespread, common and dangerous diseases was in decline long before the use of antibiotics to treat them or the use of mass vaccinations to prevent them.

Why a study has shown that only 3.5% of the decline in mortality from infectious diseases can be attributed to drug treatments.

Why approximately 6 times more men with prostate cancer who had their prostate gland surgically removed, die within 15_years of other causes, such as other cancers and heart disease.

Why, in the last 20 years, not a single study has shown that aggressive biomedical treatments for prostate cancer such as radiotherapy, although often accompanied by severe and chronic side effects and/or leading to impotence and incontinence, improve survival rates at all.

Why a participant in the Manhattan project and leading medical researcher on the effects of radiation came to believe that the use of radiotherapy for both diagnosis and treatment is "a highly important cause (probably the principal cause) of cancer mortality in the United States during the twentieth century."

Why chemotherapy for all types of cancer is still used even though it has been shown by countless reports and admitted by many cancer specialists to be ineffective even in increasing life expectancy, and why death rates from cancer have actually increased with the increased use of chemotherapy.

Why, despite the Nobel Prize winning 'discovery' that the 'cause' of stomach ulcers was not 'stress' but a specific bacterium, it was then found that between one and two-thirds of the world population carry this bacterium in their stomachs without developing ulcers.

Why 20-40% of children and 10% of adults carry the tuberculosis bacillus without contracting tuberculosis, and why only a minority of those exposed to the bacillus will develop TB.

Why children allergic to household dust at home showed no allergic responses when this dust was distributed in the hospital rooms.

Why Whitehall civil servants who are given orders by their superiors have twice the chance of contracting diabetes than those who give them their orders.

Why emotional stress tests for arterial problems in women are far more likely to reveal problems than physical stress tests.

Why counselling for cardiac patients can prevent recurrence of heart attacks or even reverse arterial blockages, and why half of all heart attacks occur in people with normal cholesterol levels.

Why patients whose surgeons talk to them whilst under anaesthesia are at less risk of dying, and why patients whose surgeons openly discuss post-operative pain before surgery experience it less.

Why someone with sensitive skin can work for years with materials they are sensitive too, and yet only develop allergic reactions when emotional problems in their relational life flare up.

Why X-rayed blood samples taken from depressed subjects had a reduced capacity for repair of cellular DNA.

Why soldiers whose armies suffered defeat in battle were more likely to develop dysentery or typhus.

Why autopsies of thousands of young and otherwise healthy soldiers revealed atherosclerotic plaques of the sort generally associated only with older people, long-term smokers and others thought to be at risk of heart attacks and strokes from developing these plaques over time.

Why 'placebos' or fake surgery can be just as effective as 'active' drugs and real surgery.

Why it is that people smoke, take illegal drugs, over- or under-eat, or *do any of the things* supposed to be a major cause of their illness.

Why off-the-counter medications and legally prescribed drugs are a cause of greater and more widespread addiction – and often more difficult to come off – than illegal drugs.

Why people become obsessed with changing to or pursuing supposedly healthy 'lifestyles' through diets or fitness regimes - yet without ever really examining their lives as such and the health of their human relationships.

Why there is hardly a single class of pharmaceutical medication that doesn't have as a possible or even common 'side effect', a short- or long-term worsening of the symptoms it was prescribed for.

Why the majority of patients seen by doctors are made up by what are called 'the worried well' – people who really need caring help and attention from someone for their life problems.

Why doctors will always ask patients 'how long' they have had a particular symptom but almost never ask *when* it started and what had been going in the patient's life at that time – or in the days, weeks, months or years before the symptom appeared.

Acknowledgements to *Why People Get Ill?* by Darian Leader and Michael Cornfield, Hamish Hamilton 2007, for several of the examples included here.

The Failure of Biomedicine to Explain Pain

One of the most important aspects of illness that biological medicine can't explain is *pain*. The standard model of pain is called *nociception* and those neurons that 'detect' pain are called 'nociceptors'. This terminology is relatively new – in the past one spoke of 'pain receptors'. This term was abandoned because of its all too obvious questionability. For how can neurons pick up or respond to pain when pain itself is essentially a *subjective experience*. So in place of 'pain receptors' neurologists speak now of 'nociceptors', a term derived from the Latin *noci* (meaning 'hurt') and emphasise that what these receptors 'detect' is not actually pain as we experience it subjectively but actual or potential *injury* or *damage* to external or internal tissue and organs. As for how the actual subjective experience of pain comes about, this is explained by the nociceptors transmitting signals to the brain via the spinal column. The brain then responds by 'allowing' or 'producing' a subjective experience of pain. Yet how the brain can produce a subjective experience *of any sort* – in this case pain – is left unexplained by this 'explanation'. Instead, the nature of the unanswered question implicit in the old idea of 'pain receptors' is simply reversed, i.e. instead of having to explain how a neuron can detect a subjective experience such as pain, what is now left unexplained is how it can *create* such an experience. Instead the model of nociception rests on the wholly unsupported and dogmatic assumption of biomedicine that conscious experiencing is an exclusive product or property of nerve tissue and the nervous system and brain, not least given that *all* bodily tissue is regarded by biomedicine as basically *insentient*. Moreover, what is *implicit* in this model is that the true 'source' of pain is not wherever you *actually feel it in your body* but precisely where you *don't and cannot feel it* – in the brain. Thus the pain you actually feel in your toe after stubbing it, for example, is, according to this model, nothing but a *subjective illusion* created by the brain through a neural mechanism. Yet the neurological concept of 'nociception' remains to this day, the standard physiological and biomedical model for the 'scientific' explanation of pain. It is so, however, despite the fact that:

1. It is counter-intuitive, running contrary to our lived experience of the source and site of pain.
2. It offers no explanation at all of how the brain can produce a subjective experience of pain.
3. It is premised on the idea that pain is a consequence of physical injury or damage, and so cannot explain why, for example: "...about 65% of soldiers who are severely wounded in battle and 20% of civilians who undergo major surgery report feeling little or no pain for hours or days after the injury or incision."[1]
4. It does not explain why "...no apparent injury can be detected in 70% of people who suffer from chronic low back pain..."[1].
5. It does not explain why even the most acute of pains can spontaneously arise and then subside without *any identifiable physiological change occurring.*
6. It does not explain why hypnosis can alleviate or even completely eliminate pain without any physical, pharmaceutical or surgical intervention – even to the point of faciliating entirely *pain-free surgery* without any use of anaesthetics.

7. It does not explain acute, chronic or recurring symptoms of muscle pain (myalgia) or nerve pain (neuralgia) for example in the form of fibromyalgia, or of facial and trigeminal neuralgia – where there is often no evidence of damage to muscle tissue or to the nerves or nerve sheaths.

8. It does not explain many forms of common pain – for example particular types of headache with no clearly identifiable physical cause. Seeing them as a result of 'stress' does not explain why someone leading a generally stressful life should experience just one particular type of pain (or any other illness symptom) or why they do so at a particular time or times and not others.

Points 3 and 7 present just a few of *many examples* in which – contrary to and in a way wholly unexplained by the standard physiological theory of pain – either injury occurs *without pain* or pain is experienced *without injury*.

Just as biomedicine seeks to 'explain' illness without first of all asking or seeking to 'explicate' what 'illness' or 'disease' essentially *is*, so also does it seek to 'explain' pain without first of all asking the most basic question of all – what essentially *is* 'pain'? Yet as Martin Heidegger points out:

"All explanation reaches only so far as the explication of that which is to be explained..." [my stress]
So: *"What good is all explaining if what has to be explained remains unclear?"*[2]

Pain is a perfect example of the *basic philosophical quandry* of biomedicine as such - namely the failure of all its explanations of illness to address and incorporate its subjective dimension, and the chicken-egg question this gives rise to: is the felt *subjective* experience of 'dis-ease' (of 'feeling ill') a mere effect of 'being ill' – of having some 'objective' physiological disease or disorder? Or could it be that it is the other way round? This is the same basic question that is avoided in biomedical explanations of pain. For whereas in ordinary language we speak of painful life experiences or conflicts and of feeling emotionally 'hurt' in all sorts of ways, biomedical science discards this everyday language of life for neurological terminologies and explanations which seek to reduce pain to an effect of purely 'physical' or 'physiological' phenomena – yet without any explanation of how the *subjective* experience of pain arises from them. Indeed simply by turning the pain into an *object* of scientific or medical explanations, biomedicine implicitly *rules out in advance* any attempt to explicate the essentially *subjective* character of pain and instead turns this into a mere 'secondary' phenomenon arising from purely 'objective' neurological mechanisms.

"The idea of one basis for science and another for life is from the very outset a lie." Karl Marx

A purely biomedical and physiological approach to pain denies it any intrinsic meaning or healthy purpose. Yet pain can serve many important purposes besides registering actual or potential tissue damage.

Examples:

- Allowing long-standing or acutely painful emotions or emotional conflicts – inner pain - to be experienced in a more intense bodily way and thus brought to a focus through a painful bodily condition or state.
- Allowing an otherwise only vaguely or dimly experienced bodily sense of dis-ease in one's life to become sharper and more acutely or intensely felt.
- Allowing the individual to indirectly *communicate* their otherwise unexpressed or inexpressible inner pain to others – for example through grimacing and groaning, contortions of the face, writhing of the body and/or 'screaming with pain'.
- Seeking in this way some form of caring recognition or empathic response from others to this inner pain.

All these purposes of pain serve to prevent not just the human body but the *human being* from suffering on-going or further 'damage'. Conversely, even where pain *is* related to actual tissue damage, this may be because it is the only way the individual is currently able to more fully experience, express and communicate their inner pain. This is also the reason why some individuals engage in intentional and conscious self-harm – seeking a temporary sense of release from an inner pain that plagues them by hurting their bodies and through sensations of physical pain. On the other hand, a period of intense physical pain may also occur just after *after* the painful life issues behind it have been resolved – offering a sense of final cathartic release from them. It is as if the individual gives themselves *permission* to experience the full intensity of an inner pain somatically after its inner alleviation. Here somatic pain serves a different type of symbolic or even ritual purpose. The extraction of a painful tooth, for example, may serve as an important external symbol and ritual for the individual – signifying and reassuring them that a source of inner pain in their lives has indeed now been finally 'removed'.

By simply shunting off both painful life experiences and 'emotional pain' into a second and entirely *separate domain* of psychology or neuropsychiatry however, the biomedical explanation of pain is classically *dualistic* – not just separating 'mind and body', the 'psychic' and the 'physical', but also and above all separating *life itself* from what is claimed to be a true account (*logos*) or 'science' of life (Greek *bios*) – namely what is called 'biology'. And by turning pain into an *object* of biological and neurological explanation however, not only does biomedicine entirely fail to explain its subjective essence, it also 'shoots itself in the foot' when it comes to treating pain – to so-called 'pain control' or 'pain management'. For it is not just doctors but also their patients who turn their own subjective pain into an *object* – into something they 'have'. This however, is unfortunate for the patient and pain sufferer – because the very bearability of pain and our capacity to live with it depends principally on our capacity to *be the pain* we experience rather than experiencing it as some thing or 'object' affecting us. 'Being the pain' – *becoming it* – is the most effective way to stop experiencing pain as some sort of bodily entity or object *separate* from our self and therefore 'causing' us to *suffer* in a way over which we actually have *no control* at all *except* through medication. 'Being the pain' means identifying with the pure *awareness* of it – an awareness which is *not itself* anything painful. Indeed actively choosing to *intensify* that awareness of pain – even the most acute of pains – can, paradoxically, alleviate our suffering as well as releasing insights into its source in our lives (see Case Example 1).

From the perspective of Life Medicine, pain is first and foremost an experience of the subjectively experienced or 'lived' body and not the so-called 'physical' body or any of its organs, not least the brain. For if the assumptions of 'brain science' itself are followed to their logical conclusion, what we perceive from the outside as the human physical body and its internal organs – including the shape and form of the brain itself – is ultimately but a subjective perceptual 'phantasm' constructed and projected outwards *by* the brain. This is the sort of philosophical *reductio ad absurdum* to which, as Heidegger indicated, 'reductionist' brain science ultimately leads – both in general and in relation to pain. For taken to its ultimate conclusion we end up with a worldview in which there is nothing we perceive or experience that can count as real except the brain, even though, paradoxically, our very perception of that organ we call 'the brain' is, according to neurological models of perception itself, nothing but a construction of the brain. Despite these philosophical paradoxes we see an increasing flood of media propaganda for so-called 'brain science' – a science that identifies who we are as human beings with our brains is evidence for this – and a useful prop for manufacturers of brain-altering drugs, including what can be highly addictive analgesics or 'pain killers'. The term itself is an interesting one – akin to the term 'killer cells' or the notion of 'fighting illness'. In contrast we have the following words of Seth and of Ivan Illich taken from the appendices of this book.

"... pain and suffering are also obviously vital, living sensations – and therefore are a part of the body's repertoire of possible feelings and sensual experience. They are also a sign, therefore, of life's vitality, and are in themselves often responsible for a return to health when they act as learning communications." Seth (from appendix 1)

"A myriad virtues express the different aspects of fortitude that traditionally enabled people to recognize painful sensations as a challenge and to shape their own experience accordingly. Patience, forbearance, courage, resignation, self-control, perseverance, and meekness each express a different colouring of the responses with which pain sensations were accepted, transformed into the experience of suffering and endured. Duty, love, fascination, routines, prayer, and compassion were some of the means that enabled pain to be borne with dignity." Illich (from appendix 3)

The pupils of Hippocrates distinguished many kinds of disharmony, each of which caused its own type of pain...Pain might disappear in the process of healing, but this was certainly not the primary object of the ... treatment. The Greeks did not even think about enjoying happiness without taking pain in their stride ... The body had not yet been divorced from the soul, nor had sickness been divorced from pain. All words that indicated bodily pain were equally applicable to the suffering of the soul." Illich (from appendix 3)

Other references:

1. Melzack and Wall, *The Challenge of Pain*, Hardmondsworth: Penguin Books, 1982
2. Heidegger, Martin *Zollikon Seminars,* Northwestern University Press, 2001

Postscript: a brief case of headache

A client complained about a having bad headache at the beginning of a session with her therapist and just before she was about to go on holiday with her partner. Asked when the headache had started she reported having woken up feeling fine but then worrying about the holiday. This was because she had promised her partner not to take any work-related books with her, knowing he was afraid that reading them would preoccupy her for too much of their time together. However, whilst packing before the session she had realised that she really would like to take at least a couple of her books along with her – but also felt bound by the promise she had made to her partner not to do so. In other words it was the inner pain, fear and guilt about a desire whose result might be to hurt her partner that triggered the headache. When her therapist suggested that she might resolve this relational dilemma by indeed taking a couple of books with her – but at the same time resolving not to get lost in reading them at the expense of spending time with her partner – she immediately realised that this could indeed offer a practical way of *reconciling* her desire not to hurt or cause pain to her partner with her equally sincere wish to enjoy at least some time reading her books. When she came to a decision in the session to follow this suggestion and to also share and negotiate a new compromise and new promise with her partner she became aware that her headache had totally disappeared.

Getting Ill to See a Doctor

"The doctor is the drug."

"...the drug 'doctor' is a potent one with many unwanted side effects."

Michael Balint

In a society in which biological medicine or 'biomedicine' is institutionally dominant and 'mental illness' is still tainted by stigma, getting ill and seeing a doctor remains the principle *socially acceptable way* for people who are consciously or unconsciously ill-at-ease with their lives to obtain the care and attention they need or seek.

Precisely for this reason however, a *primary purpose* of illness can be to serve as a *principal communicative medium* by which individuals seek – through the clinical encounter with a physician – acknowledgement of their *existential* dis-ease or *life* suffering – one whose origin or 'etiology' does not lie in the biological life of the patient's body but rather in their *life as such* and their *life-world as a whole* (including their work world, family world etc).

However the *pre-condition* demanded by the clinical encounter for attaining the acknowledgement, care and attention that the patient seeks for their existential dis-ease is that they 'present' the physician with bodily symptoms that can be neatly fitted in the diagnostic schema of biomedicine, i.e., acknowledged as signs of recognised *diseases* for which standard biomedical tests and treatments can be prescribed. If this pre-condition is *not* fulfilled the individual risks being classed as a hypochondriac, malingerer or 'heart-sink' patient, i.e., one whose symptoms, old or new, consistently defy any form of straightforward clinical diagnosis, despite repeated visits to their doctor, multiple medical tests or appointments with specialist consultants.

For the individual *not* merely to be written off or classed as a hypochondriac or malingerer, *their own body knows full well* that it must translate or 'body forth' their existential dis-ease and life suffering in the form of symptoms of an 'actual' biological illness or disease capable of diagnostic identification and treatment.

The word 'iatrogenic' comes from the Greek words *genesis* and *iatros* (physician) and is used to refer to illnesses resulting from medical treatment itself. The intrinsically *iatrogenic* dimension of biological medicine lies in the fact that in many cases *patients do not simply go to doctors because they are ill.* Instead *they become ill in order to be able to go to doctors* – to create opportunities through the clinical encounter for the indirect communication and acknowledgment of their existential dis-ease and life suffering. This is perhaps the chief purpose and meaning of illness in the context of the clinical encounter.

Particularly in the case of individuals who are lonely or isolated, or whose communicative world or abilities do not fulfil their need to be understood, the clinical encounter with a physician is sought as something *intrinsically healing* – healing simply because of the opportunity it offers for a *tiny dose of understanding communication* – however medically distorted this 'understanding' may be and however absurdly time-limited the communication itself (in contrast, for example, to a 50 minute psychotherapy session).

It is the *modicum* of human contact provided by the clinical encounter with the physician or the human care provided by hospitalisation that is most healing for the patient. In this context, it would be most interesting to have available statistics showing the number of patients whose symptoms diminish or even disappear on the *very day* of an appointment with a doctor – feeling better simply through the expectation or experience of being able to *communicate* their suffering with a human being who is, by profession, duty bound to give them care and attention, take their suffering seriously and 'understand' it – even if only in biomedical terms.

Ivan Illich identified three types of iatrogenesis – clinical, social and cultural.

'Iatrogenesis is clinical when pain, sickness and death result from medical care; it is social when health policies reinforce an industrial organization that generates ill-health; it is cultural and symbolic when medically sponsored behaviour and delusions restrict the vital autonomy of people by undermining their competence in growing up, caring for each other, and aging, or when medical intervention cripples personal responses to pain, disability, impairment, anguish and death.'

To the three types of iatrogenesis identified and described by Illich one could add a fourth. I call this 'communicative iatrogenesis'.

Communicative iatrogenesis arises from the fact that the required *language* necessary to seek and attain understanding communication through doctoring is the language of bodily *illness itself*. For whilst it would not be usual for a recently bereaved and lonely widow(er) to see a doctor in order to complain of being 'heart-broken' or of 'losing heart' to live, what *is* culturally acceptable – if not normative – is to go to a doctor and complain of pains in the region of the heart or heart arrhythmias. This is something that the patient knows. Yet – and this is the key factor – it is also something that the patient's *body* knows and is capable of responding to – by generating chest pains or heart arrhythmias. Of course there is such a thing now as 'bereavement counselling'. Yet how many prospective patients are informed or would be inclined to take it up – rather than seeing the very need for such counselling as a sign of emotional weakness.

Communicative iatrogenesis can be understood as a fundamental dimension of what Illich himself calls 'cultural and symbolic' iatrogenesis – biomedically diagnosable illness being a culturally determined and also symbolic *password* for obtaining the sought-after acknowledgement and communication of an individual's life suffering *through* that illness and in the *context* of the clinical encounter.

From this perspective, the 'ordinary' patient is just as much an individual in need of and in search of attention, care and communicative understanding as the 'heart-sink patient' or 'hypochondriac'. The distinction lies in the fact that the latter may ultimately fail to fulfil their needs through the clinical encounter. This is because they lack the central 'key' to obtaining the critical 'password' to it. This key is their willingness to *let* their own body translate or 'body forth' their existential disease or life suffering – not just in the form of medical *symptoms* but in the form of a 'genuine' – medically diagnosable – biological illness or disease.

In considering the origin or 'etiology' of illness from an existential and 'hermeneutic' perspective therefore – one that focuses on the *meaning* and *purpose* of illness rather than its biological 'causes' – we cannot exclude *the existential meaning of the clinical encounter for the patient* and the *purpose that illness serves within its* biomedical framework, i.e., as a necessary 'password' to that encounter and the opportunity it offers for fulfilling basic communicative needs.

The idea that becoming ill has a *meaning and purpose* is heretical enough in a cultural climate dominated by biological medicine. The sad paradox is that in such a culture the relational healing that patients seek through fulfilment of their basic human needs – for human contact, care and understanding communication – can be met only by getting *physically ill*. Thus whilst children are often understood to complain of symptoms or even to somehow 'actually' get ill as a way of seeking attention, the culture of biomedicine demands that *adults* do the same thing – simply in order to *call attention* to their existential dis-ease, their life suffering, stress or distress.

The Medical Consultation as a 'Set Up'

A patient wishes to *make sense* of his or her symptoms and arranges to see a doctor. So an appointment is duly made. Yet what remains unspoken in the consultation is that it is tacitly expected to take as its starting point certain unquestioned assumptions which serve as expected 'points of departure' for all doctor-patient communication. Below I list some of the most basic tacit assumptions that 'enframe' the medical consultation and constitute expected points of departure for all communication that occurs within it.

1. It is tacitly understood that we all know what 'illness' and 'health' are, that they are opposites, and that 'illness' is something 'bad' and 'health' something 'good'.

2. It is tacitly understood and agreed that the patient arranges the consultation because he is suffering symptoms of a possible 'illness' which he wishes to have identified and which he or she is therefore prepared to have diagnosed through examination and testing and be prescribed treatment for.

3. It is tacitly understood and agreed that the patient will describe their symptoms and that the physician will, directly or through further tests, arrive at a medical diagnosis of the disease, recommend a course of biomedical treatment aimed at relieving their symptoms or 'curing' the disease – based on knowledge of its biological 'causes'.

4. It is tacitly understood and agreed that the patient has just happened to fall victim to their symptoms 'out of the blue' – in other words that there is no meaning to be attached to the specific timing of their appearance in the larger context of the patient's life and life history.

5. It is tacitly understood and agreed therefore, that symptoms have no meaning at all beyond being mere signs of a possible biological disease or dysfunction.

6. It is tacitly understood and agreed therefore that 'making sense' of symptoms means nothing more than taking them as possible signs of some biomedical disease – and that in no case can a biological illness or disease be itself taken as a symptom of a life-disease – a hidden life problem that manifests in the patient feeling 'ill-at-ease' with their lives.

7. It is tacitly understood and agreed that the patient's suffering – their felt pain, discomfort or 'dis-ease' – is a mere secondary and subjective 'effect' of an organic disorder or 'disease'. The contrary notion, namely that symptoms, illness and disease may be a symbolic embodiment of a subjectively felt dis-ease' – and of particular ways in which the patient is 'ill-at-ease' with their life – is ruled out in advance. Indeed such a notion constitutes sheer heresy in terms of the unquestioned dogmas of biomedical 'science'.

Should a patient reject any or all of these assumptions, or depart from any of the unspoken rules or points of departure in their communication with a doctor, the patient will be immediately classed as a 'difficult' or 'incompliant' patient or even as deluded. Yet together these tacitly agreed assumptions and points of departure for a biomedical consultation effectively constitute an unspoken 'set up' or 'frame up' – a framework the patient is expected to compliantly adhere to. The aim of this 'frame up' is to enframe the meaning of the patient's symptoms in the terms of one framework only – that of biomedicine – excluding any other possible ways of making sense of those symptoms. Any attempt by a patient to question this framework – even if only by not immediately accepting certain types of routine biomedical tests or courses of treatment – will arouse indignation and bewilderment, be seen as a threat to the authority of bio-medically trained doctors and a waste of the limited time they give to their patients. Instead it could be seen as an opportunity to give themselves more time to learn about the lives of their patients as human beings, to understand their symptoms in the larger context of their life and life world.

What Most Doctors Don't Ask

What follows is a list of some of the questions that most doctors don't ask – and yet which are key questions for both doctor and patient in coming to understand the life meaning of particular symptoms. They are the sort of questions central to Life Medicine and Life Doctoring – those that a Life Doctor will always begin by asking and discussing with the patient.

When did your symptoms first occur?

What was going on in your life in the hours, days, weeks, months or years preceding the onset of your symptoms?

What were the most significant life encounters, events, experiences, dilemmas and decisions that faced you in the period preceding the onset of your symptoms?

Was there any sort of underlying or overall mood you experienced in this period and how would you describe it?

What were the most dominant thoughts and emotions you experienced in this period?

What thoughts tend to accompany your symptoms?

What feelings tend to accompany these thoughts?

How to you respond to these thoughts and feelings when they arise, and how do they affect your symptoms?

What beliefs do you hold about your symptoms and the right way to respond to them?

What do you tend to do in response to your symptoms themselves?

At what specific times or in what specific life situations do your symptoms tend to occur, recur or increase in intensity or frequency?

At what times or in what situations do your symptoms tend to disappear, diminish or reduce in frequency?

Have you experienced similar symptoms in the past, and if so at what times and in what circumstances?

How do your symptoms, and the thoughts and feelings you have around them, affect your life, work and relationships?

What do the symptoms force you to do, stop you doing or allow you to do?

Is there any positive benefit you can see from the way your symptoms affect your life?

How would you describe the overall or underlying mood or state of consciousness accompanying your symptoms and/or the thoughts and emotions around them?

How do your symptoms make *you* feel? In what way does the mood that accompanies them affect not only *what* you think and *how* you feel but also *who* you are - your sense of 'you'?

Is there any positive side to the different mood and sense of self accompanying your symptoms and/or to what they force or give you permission to do – or not to do?

Are there any other ways in which you could give expression in your life to this positive and healthy side of the symptoms – without needing those symptoms as a spur to do so?

Alternatively, what changes in your life world or way of relating to life and other people do you feel would most help to alter this underlying mood and/or alleviate your symptoms?

What are the most important types of experience you miss or have missed in your life and relationships?

What are the most important potentials or abilities you feel are not or have not been fulfilled or realised in your life?

What do you see as the most important life events or experiences you have had?

What do you see as the most important life turning points or life decisions you have made?

Were there particular dilemmas associated with or generated by these life events or experiences, turning points or decisions – and if so what were they?

Making Things Worse
through Medication

(see also appendix on *Death by Doctoring*)

"...serious reactions to prescription drugs are responsible for 250,000 Britons being hospitalised each year – with aspirin, diuretics, warfarin and NSAIDs (non-steroidal anti-inflammatory drugs arthritis the main offenders." Ben Ong

Millions of prescriptions for highly profitable drugs are handed out each year by doctors – even though the 'clinical trials' which made them available often show them to be barely more effective than placebos. At the same time, sales of over-the-counter (OTC) drugs such as pain killers bring in equally huge profits – despite often leading to chronic dependency. The counter-productivity of their possible side effects (doing the very opposite of what they are prescribed for) and the often severe and chronic withdrawal symptoms generated by different classes of common legal drug medications is shown below – using information from the makers and users of these drugs, together with the 'small print' in the instructions and warnings to patients that come with them. Just as the price paid for drug medications is kept artificially high by clever marketing – so also does the price paid by the body for using them continue to rise.

Drug class: ANXIOLYTICS (a new name for tranquilisers)
Side effects and/or withdrawal symptoms – *addiction leading to acute and chronic anxiety, irritability and restlessness, panic attacks, seizures, chronic sleep difficulties and/or muscular tension*

Drug class: SLEEPING PILLS such as temazepam
Side effects and/or withdrawal symptoms: *chronic rebound insomnia, nightmares, premature deaths (up to 500,000 in the U.S. alone according to the British Medical Journal Open Journal).*

Drug class: ANTIDEPRESSANTS (SSRI-type such as Seroxat/Paxil/Prozac)
Side effects and/or withdrawal symptoms – *depressive or manic symptoms, suicidal thoughts, suicide, aggressive behaviour, extreme violence*

Drug class: ANALGESICS (prescription or OTC pain killers and headache pills such as codeine or paracetemol)
Side effects and/or withdrawal symptoms – *nausea, digestive problems, chronic or recurrent rebound headaches.*

Drug class: ANTIINFLAMMATORY drugs such as Ibuprofen used for conditions such as arthritis
Side effects: doubling the risk of strokes and miscarriage.

Drug class: ANTICONVULSANTS (for epilepsy, nerve pain and seizures)
Side effects or withdrawal symptoms – *seizures*

Drug class: ANTIBIOTICS (for bacterial infections)
Side effects and/or withdrawal symptoms: *increased susceptibility to infection from increasingly resistant bacteria*

Drug class: PRESCRIPTION SKIN CREAMS (for skin disorders or infections)
Side effects: *acute or chronic skin damage and disorders, infections or inflammations*

Drug class: STATINS (for reducing cholesterol and protecting from heart attacks & strokes)
Side effects: *muscle weakness, fatigue, heart attacks, shortness of breath or difficulty breathing, strokes and death*

Drug class: BIPHOSPHATE BONE DRUGS (for osteoporosis and brittle bones)
Side effects: *increased risk of bone fracture*

Drug class: DIET PILLS
Side effects: depression, suicidal ideation, suicide

Drug class: ANTI-SMOKING PILLS
Side effects: suicide, suicidal thoughts, depression, nausea and vomiting

Drug class: VACCINES
Side effects: *increased susceptibility to infection (for example to flu, measles, polio etc.)*

EXAMPLE: below is a list of side effects included in the maker's own patient information leaflet for a skin cream currently prescribed for skin infections, reddening, swelling and itchiness and a variety of other skin conditions and disorders.

LISTED SIDE EFFECTS: *Severe rash, burning and stinging feeling, skin irritation, itching skin, worsening of your eczema, thinning of the skin, small veins near the surface of the skin become visible, stretch marks, itchy rash and skin inflammation in the area where the medicine is used, red spotting rash around the mouth or chin, skin of the face may become puffy, irritation to the eyes and mucus membranes (such as lips or genital area).*

How Biomedical Diagnosis
can Damage Your Health

Diagnostic screening

"Diagnosis may exclude a human being with 'bad' genes from being born, another from promotion, and a third from political life. The mass hunt for health risks begins with dragnets designed to apprehend those needing special protection … Health testing … was welcomed as the poor man's escalator into the world of Mayo [the Mayo Clinic] and Massachusetts General … [yet] studies indicate that these diagnostic procedures – even when followed up by high-level medical treatments – have no positive impact on life-expectancy … in any case, it transforms people who feel healthy into patients anxious for their verdict."
Ivan Illich

Example: screening of men for higher than normal age-levels of PSA (Prostate Specific Antigen) of a sort which may indicate the presence of cancer of the prostate.

Diagnostic statistics

"By equating statistical man with biologically unique men, an insatiable demand for finite [medical] resources is created … the right of the patient to withhold consent to his own treatment vanishes as the doctor argues that he must submit to diagnosis, since society cannot afford the burden of curative procedures that would be even more expensive."

Example: enormous pressure is placed on men with high PSA levels to undergo intrusive needle biopsies in order to extract cell samples for analysis and confirm the presence of cancerous cells – even though such biopsies produce many 'false negative' results, and even positive results allow no firm *prognostic* conclusions to be drawn whatsoever.

That is why one reading of the acronym PSA is 'Producer of Stress and Anxiety'.

Diagnostic screening statistics

Example: Two large, long-awaited studies [reported by the New England Journal of Medicine] failed to produce convincing evidence that routine prostate-cancer screening significantly reduces the chances of dying from the disease without putting men at risk for potentially dangerous and unnecessary treatment. The PSA blood test, which millions of men undergo each year, did not cut the death toll from the disease in the first decade of a U.S. government-funded study involving more than 76,000 men, researchers reported yesterday.

In the U.S. study, researchers randomly assigned 76,693 men ages 55 to 74 at 10 centres to receive either six annual screenings consisting of PSA testing and physical examinations or whatever their doctors recommend, which could include screening.

After seven years, 22 percent more prostate cancers were diagnosed in the PSA group, and 17 percent more were diagnosed after 10 years. But there was no significant difference in deaths from the cancer in the two groups. The researchers noted there were actually more deaths overall in the screened group – 312 vs. 225 – and they could not rule out that the excess may have been the result of overtreatment.

The second study, a European trial involving more than 162,000 men that was released simultaneously, did find fewer deaths among those tested. But the reduction was relatively modest, and the study showed that the screening resulted in a large number of men undergoing needless, often harmful treatment.

Rob Stein, Philadelphia Inquirer, 2009

Diagnostic stress and isolation

"Diagnosis always intensifies stress, defines incapacity, imposes inactivity, and focuses apprehension on non-recovery, on uncertainty and on one's dependence on future medical findings, all of which amounts to a loss of autonomy ... It also isolates a person in a special role, separates him from the normal and healthy, and requires submission to the authority of specialised personnel. Once a society organises for a preventative disease-hunt, it gives epidemic proportions to diagnosis. This ultimate triumph of therapeutic culture turns the independence of the average healthy person into an intolerable form of deviance."
Ivan Illich

Example: the diagnosis of prostate cancer – like any form of cancer – produces an unhealthy degree of anxiety and stress, fear and uncertainty of a sort which makes the individual more likely to passively submit to medical authority and with it to dangerous and damaging forms of further diagnostic testing and/or treatments such as chemo- or radio-therapy – all of which, in the case of prostate cancer, drastically reduce quality of life whilst bringing no definitive 'cure' and often requiring further repeated and debilitating treatments.

Diagnostic error

"Diagnostic bias in favour of sickness combines with frequent diagnostic error. Medicine not only imputes questionable categories with inquisitorial enthusiasm; it does so at a rate of miscarriage that no court system could tolerate. In one instance, autopsies showed that more than half the patients who died in a British university clinic with a diagnosis of specific heart failure had in fact died of something else." (Illich, ibid.)

Example: many men die *with* prostate cancer even though they have not died from it.

Diagnostic damage and 'iatrogenesis'

Example: many forms of diagnostic testing are potentially dangerous and damaging in themselves. In the case of prostate cancer biopsies they not only accentuate the very symptoms that first led them to be done (e.g. urinary difficulties, production of blood in the urine) or produce infections of the prostate. Should cancerous cells be found, the biopsy procedure itself increases the likelihood of these cells spreading to other parts of the body – thus helping to realise the worst possible outcome and prognosis of a malignant tumour through the very procedure of diagnosis itself. In this way diagnosis itself becomes a form of *iatrogenesis* – medically generated disease. As for actual treatments of prostate cancer, in a large proportion of cases these can result not only in the generally debilitating effects of such therapies but also in permanent impotence.

Biomedicine as
Money-Driven Medicine

The increasing trend toward the privatisation of medicine has its roots in the privatisation of illness *as such* – and in the massive corporate profits that can be derived therefrom.

Yet to reduce illness to the private property of an individual's body is to wholly ignore the role played in illness by the *sickness of the world and planet* they live in – whether in the form of economic deprivation, ecological destruction, environmental poisoning and – last but not least, worldwide wars.

Then again, endless political debates about how to deal with the ever-increasing costs of funding for national or private health provision all fail to get the central point – namely, that in capitalist economies, the medical diagnosis and treatment of illness is essentially *big business* and *money-driven* – exploited for the promotion of new medical drugs and technologies. That is why the big pharmaceutical companies make more profits than all the Fortune 500 corporations put together.

What is conventionally regarded as 'science-based' or 'evidence-based' medicine is actually *nothing of the sort* – given the corners cut by Big Pharma in testing new drugs, in informing the public on their true and often minimal efficacy, in warning them of their side-effects and often serious dangers – not to mention the massive sums of money spent *not* on costly 'R&D' but purely on marketing the latest drugs and treatments to doctors and surgeons. Even the most reputable medical professionals and 'experts' are now regularly paid to have articles offering misleading 'evidence' for the efficacy and 'safety' of new drugs and medical technologies published in their name – whether or not they have participated in that research or even so much as read the articles sent for their signature. In reality, modern medicine and its treatments have been acknowledged by the *Journal of the American Medical Association* itself to be *the third leading cause of death* after cancer and diabetes.

Money-driven medicine has effectively turned patients themselves into commodities for sale by their physicians – offering a source of profit not just through drugs but through expensive hi-tech testing and 'treatment' technologies. All this at massive expense to national health services and/or to the profit of private health providers milking health insurance companies or even public health services.

The truth is that illness is essentially big business, that 'Big Pharma is Big Bucks and Bad Medicine', and that today's 'evidence-based' medicine is essentially Money-Driven Medicine. Indeed any drug or new medical technology that actually 'cured' a disease would be fatal for the profits of the entire Medical-Industrial Complex. Nevertheless the *promise* of cure is constantly promoted by this multi-trillion dollar medical industry - one with vast lobbying power and almost complete monetary control of regulatory organisations such as the Food and Drug Administration in the U.S.A.

"The pharmaceutical companies have become the favourite whipping boy in discussions about the corrupting influence of money in medicine. And the companies deserve a lot of the criticism they receive ... but I want to be clear that they are not the only problem. The larger truth is that creating new patients and making more diagnoses benefits an entire medical-industrial complex that includes Pharma but also manufacturers of medical devices and diagnostic technologies, *freestanding diagnostic centers, surgical centers, and even academic medical centers."*

Dr. H. Gilbert Welch, *Over-Diagnosed – making people sick in the pursuit of health*

To put it bluntly, there are surely understandable *reasons* for people feeling or even getting seriously anxious, depressed or sick if they can't earn a living wage, can't rent or pay for housing, if their homes are threatened with foreclosure, if they face a daily threat of joblessness – or can see no chance of realising their life potentials. Yet modern 'scientific' medicine consistently ignores such reasons for both mental and physical illnesses, instead reducing them to a result of chemical imbalances in the brain or biological 'causes' of one sort or another. In this way it totally denies all *life-meaning* to illness – and its relation to the innate sickness and sickness-generating effects of capitalism itself.

Complementary medicine and proponents of alternative psychosomatic, psychoanalytic and existential understandings of illness frequently either ignore or downplay its social, political and economic dimensions. For capitalism also profits from illness in another way - by manufacturing it on an industrial scale through the dis-ease generated by what Marx called wage-slavery. This is the prostitution of the individuals' 'labour power' i.e. their bodies – to make profits for an employer, only for the employee to be casually disposed of through unemployment at times of economic downturn.

Yet what 'employment' itself means in capitalism is that anyone from skilled and experienced workers, to unemployed graduates, budding artists, musicians or scientists whose education or training, skills, interests and actual *work* has no current 'market value' can be forced into employment in the form of any low-paid job offered to them, even if it doesn't pay them a minimum or living wage – or in no way actually 'employs' their true skills, gifts or potentials.

In these circumstances, illness can thus serve as a form of *mute political protest* at the economic demands imposed by capitalism and the distress this imposes on people. For it offers the individual time to temporarily reclaim their body as their own, and allow it to embody and symbolically register their felt dis-ease and distress in what, for most, is the only socially acceptable way – through medical disease symptoms. The problem is then that their bodies are immediately *reclaimed* by medical professionals and the medical-industrial complex, in a way that actively furthers the process of translating and transforming an individual's felt 'dis-ease' into some medically diagnosable 'disease'. The patient's body is perceived and treated as a biological machine – rather than as a living embodiment of the human being. And as with any other machine, the aim is to repair it and restore its economic functionality.

For just as capitalism identifies work solely with 'employment' that profits an employer, so also it identifies 'health' solely with an individual's economic 'functionality', i.e. the capacity for 'employment' in the labour market rather than the capacity to engage in personally meaningful activity or work – irrespective of its 'market value'. Similarly capitalism recognises as 'illness' only that which interferes with the mechanical functioning of body and mind in the performance of mechanical tasks, physical or mental. All this has recently become ever clearer through governments making receipt of welfare benefits for the dependent on tests designed only to show that (totally irrespective of the individual's medical condition and indeed even if they are terminally ill) they are still capable of *employment of some sort* – even if they can't get a job, even if that job does not pay a living wage and even if it is clearly *damaging* to both their medical health and their essential 'health' i.e. their capacity for living a meaningful and fulfilled *life*.

The role of the doctor in what is ever-more evidently a money-driven medicine is – paradoxically – to rule out entirely from consideration the larger life context in which an illness first manifests – not least its economic context and the effect of the latter on the patient's social world and relationships. Thus, loss of housing, jobs or life opportunities of the sort that lead to disheartenment and loss of heart on the part of patients count for nothing – until and unless this loss of heart manifests as diagnosable symptoms of 'heart disease'. These are then, like all other forms of illness, cold-heartedly treated as if they had nothing to do with the patient's actual life whatsoever. The role of the biomedical doctor is principally to act and do – to *treat* patients and not to talk with them - and certainly not to *listen* to them, to hear and feel their inner 'dis-ease' and learn about the health of their *lives* and relationships. The seemingly idealistic aim of improving patients' health and 'saving' or 'extending' patients' lives through medical tests and treatments of all sorts is pursued at any cost to their bodies as a result of serious side-effects and at whatever expense to their real health i.e. their *quality* of life.

The result is a veritable epidemic of 'preventative' screening – at high cost to public health services - but resulting in over-diagnosis and over-treatment, even of people with no symptoms whatsoever. This leads in turn to widespread 'iatrogenetic' (medically caused) illnesses – which then require yet further medical treatments. A prime example is screening men for prostate cancer by conducting blood tests which measure their level of 'PSA' (Prostate Specific Antigen). If this is found to be above a set figure, intrusive biopsies are then regularly conducted. These can produce the very symptoms of prostate cancer they were supposed to prevent from emerging – as well as increasing the likelihood of any actual cancer spreading through the body. Yet as many doctors admit, most men die *with* and not *from* prostate cancer – whereas surgical and drug treatments for it can and often do dramatically reduce their quality of life, for example through making them impotent or incontinent.

Constant government, media and press propaganda regarding 'health risks' of all sorts, together with mass screening programs, serve a vital role in maintaining money-driven medicine and the medical-industrial complex – creating a type of *mass hypochondria* which feeds it with new patients to be medically processed or peddled with new drugs. No better was this pathological state of affairs expressed than by Illich:

"People who are angered, sickened and impaired by their industrial labour and leisure can escape only into a life under medical supervision and are thereby seduced or disqualified from political struggle for a healthier world."

"A professional and physician-based health-care system that has grown beyond critical bounds is sickening for three reasons: it must produce clinical damage that outweighs its potential benefits; it cannot but enhance even as it obscures the political conditions that render society unhealthy; and it tends to expropriate the power of the individual to heal himself and shape his or her environment."

"More and more people subconsciously know that they are sick and tired of their jobs and of their leisure passivities, but they want to hear the lie that physical illness relieves them of social and political responsibilities. They want their doctor to act as lawyer and priest. As a lawyer, the doctor exempts the patient from his normal duties and enables him to cash in on the insurance fund he was forced to build. As a priest, he becomes the patient's accomplice in creating the myth that he is an innocent victim of biological mechanisms rather than a lazy, greedy or envious deserter of a social struggle for control over the tools of production. Social life becomes a giving and receiving of therapy: medical, psychiatric, pedagogic or geriatric."

"Medicine has the authority to label one man's complaint a legitimate illness, to declare a second man sick though he does not himself complain, and to refuse a third social recognition of his pain, his disability and even his death. For rich and poor … life is reduced to a 'span', to a statistical phenomenon which, for better or worse, must be institutionally planned and shaped. This life-span is brought into existence with the pre-natal check-up…and it will end with a mark on a chart…"

Illich, Ivan *Medical Nemesis – the Expropriation of Health*

The Focus of Biological Medicine – The Clinical Body

The focus of biological medicine is the 'clinical body'. This clinical body is not the actual body of any individual human being – not my body or yours. Instead it is a body constituted entirely by a *body of knowledge* – specifically the body of knowledge accumulated in the form of medical terms and textbooks and imparted through medical and clinical training. The 'gaze' of the physician derives entirely from this body of medical and clinical knowledge – and is directed only at the 'clinical body'. It is a purely *clinical gaze* – one which turns the body into an object of medical-scientific examination and clinical testing.

The clinical 'objectification' of the body through biological science and medicine totally separates the human body from the human being – both in theory and practice. It encourages patients to distance themselves from their own bodies and to see their illness itself as an impersonal object or thing – 'something' which is 'wrong with me' and which has come about - and can get 'better' or 'worse' – in a way that essentially has nothing to do with any 'me'. Medical treatment is seen as having the power to identify and eliminate this 'thing' and, like mummy, to 'make it go away' or 'make it better'.

The physician's interest is also in feeling that they *have* this power – the power to get rid of something, make it go away or make it better. The fact is however, that the patient's subjectively felt dis-ease, distress, discomfort or even pain is not essentially any 'thing' at all. It can no more be some 'thing' that can be found inside the patient's body than a grief-stricken heart can be found through a cardiogram or by prising open a patient's chest in surgery. And its meaning is nothing that can be measured.

"How does one measure grief? Obviously we cannot measure it at all. Why not? Were we to apply a method of measurement to grief, this would go against the meaning of grief and we would rule out in advance the grief as grief."

Martin Heidegger

Indeed, the very *space* in which the patient's dis-ease or discomfort, grief, pain or despair is felt is not itself a clinically observable, measurable, organic or physical space. Instead it is an invisible, non-physical space - comparable to the invisible inner space of *meaning* that lies behind *a word*. Yet no amount of 'scientific' knowledge, investigation or analysis of a book's 'body' of paper and chemical ink marks (or of electronic pixels on a screen of text) will ever reveal 'evidence' of the world of *meaning* its words arise from, express and communicate.

Similarly, no amount of clinical knowledge of the human body's organic structure and diseases can ever reveal 'evidence' even of the very *existence* of the human *being* whose body it is – let alone discern the larger life *meaning* of their felt dis-ease.

Through its exclusive focus on diagnosing and treating the 'clinical body', neither the individual's *felt* body, the individual human *being* – nor the individual world of *meaning* in which they live – actually *have any place in biological medicine* at all. Consequently, biological medicine – no matter how much treatment it gives to the clinical body – *cannot actually 'cure' a single human being*. Instead only the patient's illness can do that – through recognition of its meaning for the patient *as* a human being.

Reference: Foucault, Michel *The Birth of the Clinic*

PART 3
ON LIFE MEDICINE

Basic Principles of Life Medicine

- Illnesses have life *meanings* and not just biological 'causes'.

- People die *through* illnesses – not 'because' of them – and that only if they are *ready* to die.

- It is not illnesses that are the problem in our lives - but the *life problems* that express themselves as illnesses.

- The body is not a biological machine or a product of our genes but a living biological *language* of the human being.

- Health is not merely our capacity to 'function' economically in the labour market but an expression of the degree of fulfilment we experience in our lives, work and relationships.

Life Medicine is 'holistic' medicine in the truest sense, exploring the relation between the life of our bodies and our lives and life world as a whole.

Life Medicine challenges the whole separation between what is called 'physical', 'organic' or 'somatic' illness on the one hand and 'psychological' or 'mental' illness on the other.

Life Medicine is not merely 'psychosomatic' medicine – it does not merely focus on a limited category of so-called 'psychosomatic' or 'stress-related' illnesses.

Life Medicine recognises that every bodily state is at the same time a 'psychological' state or state of consciousness – and that every state of consciousness is at the same time a felt bodily state.

Life Medicine recognises that for many if not most people, illness is the only way they can give expression to and gain recognition of the ways they are *ill-at-ease* with their lives.

Life Medicine affirms the healing value of illness itself, recognising that the sense of 'not feeling ourselves' that marks the onset of symptoms can be the beginning of a journey that leads to 'feeling another self' – one that feels more at ease with ourselves and our lives.

Life Medicine understands illness as a form of pregnancy with its own gestation period and labour pains. From this perspective, illness is not just something to 'bear' or put up with. Instead its purpose – one that Life Doctoring can help to fulfil – is to help us to give birth to and embody a new bodily sense of self and a new inner bearing toward our lives and life relationships. In this sense, it can be said that *the illness is there to cure the patient* – to offer them healing insights into themselves and bring about a healing transformation in their lives.

Healing through Feeling

'Diagnosis' in Life Medicine and Life Doctoring does not mean seeking a medical label or 'cause' for one's symptoms. It means getting to know oneself in an intimate feeling way (*gnosis*) through (*dia*) one's symptoms. Illness symptoms not only 'affect' one's life and one's overall mental, emotional or somatic state. They are themselves the expression of a 'self state' or 'body identity' – a particular way of feeling oneself bodily in a particular life context or situation. Every bodily state or condition in other words, is not just something 'physical' but is at the same time a *state of consciousness* – and vice versa. It is also a 'self state' or 'body identity'. That is why through giving ourselves time to simply feel our symptoms *more* intensely rather than less – we can come to understand them in a new way – not as signs of some possible 'disease' but as symbolic expressions of a felt dis-ease relating to one or more aspect of our life – and also constituting a distinct state of consciousness, 'self state' or 'body identity' in its own right.

The key to self-healing is to feel and sense the symptoms we experience in a new way – not just as localised physical sensations or mental-emotional states however, but as self-states – as ways of feeling oneself and one's life. Any symptoms, if fully felt and followed in this way – meditated rather than medicated – will lead inevitably to healing insights into one's life and to a renewed and transformed sense of self. This is not because we are 'curing' ourselves without biomedical treatment, but because it is our very existence –

our relation to life – that is what is most essentially calling for healing.

As in the 'Process-Oriented' work of Arnold Mindell, 'healing' can take the form of actively encouraging the patient to amplify or 'aggravate' their felt sensations of pain or discomfort – to feel them more intensely or acutely rather than less. What Mindell found was that this could bring about the release of emotions, mental images and inner comprehensions that expressed the felt meaning of their symptoms. Mindell has applied this method to all types of symptoms, and to all dimensions of the patient's experience of illness – mental, emotional and somatic.

If a patient fears or wishes for death for example, he might ask them, there and then, to die – thus encouraging them to fearlessly feel and face the 'death process'. He understood also that for some patients, as in essence it is for all of us, death itself is nothing to be fought against in principle – as biological medicine does – but it is an intrinsic part of *life* and is invariably a healing in itself i.e. a way of finding life meaning and fulfilment in other dimensions of reality in ways that might be or have become impossible in an individual's physical life and existence.

Like Life Medicine, Mindell's work challenges the historic and hitherto unquestioned premise of all forms of medicine – the fundamental belief that its purpose is to treat and if possible 'cure' disease and thereby also to prolong *physical* life and the life of the *physical body*. Ideas of a 'life after death' are considered to be a mere matter of personal 'belief' rather than a scientific question – not surprisingly given that current 'science' ignores the fact that the 'soul' itself has its own innate bodily form, and that our felt body, as a *body of awareness*, is indeed also an eternal 'soul body' which, like our dream body, has its source and reality in other dimensions of awareness beyond the physical. Indeed Mindell speaks of what I term the felt body or 'lived body' – in other words our eternal *soul body* or *body of awareness* - as the 'dreambody' or 'dreaming body'.

This is a significant term for another reason. For it reflects also a deep comprehension that symptoms of illness emerge in the same way as *dreams* do and that illnesses can be understood as 'body dreams' – as embodied dreams – or nightmares. From this point of view it makes no more sense to regard sickness as an 'unnatural' deviation from a 'normal' state of health than it does to regard dreaming as an unnatural or abnormal disruption of sleep, or to regard nightmares in particular as an 'unhealthy type' of dream. The biomedical model of illness on the other hand, based as it is on the premise that illness is a *meaningless* deviation from health, is as outdated as certain pre-Freudian 'scientific' beliefs that dreams are *meaningless* discharges of neurological energy. Instead of seeing dreams as a mere function or by-product of some organ of the physical body – the brain – Life Medicine understands the so-called 'physical' body itself as an *embodiment* of our subjectively felt or lived body, itself a subjective body or body of feeling awareness – our 'soul body'. It is *this* body that we experience directly both in our dreams and after death – and that expresses itself in and as our entire dream environment and every other body we experience in it. The terms 'dream body' or 'dreaming body' thus points to a fundamental truth – namely that we do not first 'have' a physical body which we then come to feel and experience subjectively. Instead what we call 'the body' is most essentially a specific field pattern of awareness or *pattern of feeling awareness* – one which *bodies* itself in both the process of *dreaming* and through its physical embodiment in waking life.

Dreaming on the one hand, and what Heidegger called *bodying* on the other, are thus intimately connected. In dreaming we *body* our feeling awareness in non-physical forms. Conversely, in waking life we 'dream' that feeling awareness into a specific physical form. Yet our 'felt body' - our subjective feeling awareness of this 'physical' body is in reality a *distinct body of awareness in its own right* – a 'soul body' that we both manifest physically and also give manifold form to in our dreams. Hence the type of connections between dream symbols and physical symptoms that Freud was aware of and that revealed themselves in the following example of what Mindell calls 'healing through feeling' – a basic and innate capacity of our feeling awareness or 'soul' and *its* body.

Case Example 1

from *Working with the Dreaming Body* by Arnold Mindell:

"A patient with whom I was working was dying of stomach cancer. He was lying in the hospital bed, groaning and moaning in pain. Have you ever seen someone who is dying? It was really quite sad and terrifying. They flip quickly between trance states, ordinary consciousness and extreme pain. Once, when he was able to speak, he told me that the tumour in his stomach was unbearably painful. I had had an idea that we should focus on his proprioception, that is, his experience of the pain, so I told him that since he'd already been operated on unsuccessfully, we might try something new. He agreed, and so I suggested that he try to make the pain even worse.

He said he knew exactly how he could do that and told me that the pain felt like something in his stomach trying to break out. If he helped it break out, he said, the pain worsened. He lay on his back and started to increase the pressure in his stomach. He pushed his stomach out and kept pushing and pressing and exaggerating the pain until he felt as if he were going to explode. Suddenly, at the height of his pain, he said 'Oh, Arny, I just want to explode!' At that point he switched out of his body experience and began to talk to me. He told me that he needed to explode and asked if I would help him to do so. 'My problem', he said, 'is that I've never expressed myself sufficiently, and even when I do it's never enough.'

This problem is an ordinary, psychological problem that appears in many cases, but with him it became somatised and was pressing him now, urgently expressing itself in the form of a tumour. That was the end of our physical work together. He lay back and felt much better. Though he had been given only a short time to live and had been on the verge of death, his condition improved and he was discharged from the hospital. I went to see him afterwards very often, and every time he 'exploded' with me. He'd make noises, shout and scream, with absolutely no encouragement on my part.

... It was then also that I discovered the vital link between dreams and body symptoms. Shortly before he had entered the hospital, the patient dreamed that he an incurable disease and that the medicine for it was like a bomb. When I asked him about the bomb he made a very emotional sound and cried like a bomb dropping in the air, 'it goes up in the air and spins around sshhhss ... pfftfff.' At that moment I knew that the cancer was the bomb in his dream ... his body was literally exploding with pent-up expression. In this way his pain became his own medicine ...

In a flash I discovered that there must be something like a dreambody, an entity which is both dream and body at once ... The way I discovered the concept of the dreambody was through what I called amplification. I amplified my client's body, or proprioceptive experience and I amplified the exploding process which was mirrored in his dream."

The Healing Value of Illness

"...the body's symptoms are not necessarily pathological, that is, they are not just sicknesses which must be healed, repressed or cured. Symptoms are potentially meaningful and purposeful conditions. They could be the beginning of fantastic phases of life, or they could bring one amazingly close to the centre of existence. They can also be a trip into another world, as well as a royal road into the development of the personality."

Arnold Mindell

"If people become ill, it is quite fashionable to say that the immunity system has temporarily failed – yet the body itself knows that certain 'dis-eases' are healthy reactions. The body does not recognise <u>diseases as diseases</u> in usually understood terms. It regards all activity as experience, as a momentary condition of life, as a balancing situation."

Seth – from 'The Way Toward Health' by Jane Roberts

In its 'war against disease' – a war conducted at whatever cost to the state or to the individual – neither the meaning of illness nor the potentially healing value of illness are acknowledged by biological and genetic medicine. Life Medicine, on the other hand is founded on the recognition that illnesses can themselves serve many different healing purposes:

- Giving bodily expression to a felt 'dis-ease' – to ways in which we may feel ill-at-ease with ourselves, other people or different aspects of our lives.

- Forcing us to take 'time out' from merely 'functioning' in a physically or economically desired way.

- Helping us to feel, focus on and confront painful life problems – even if only through the way in which physical pain can itself focus the mind.

- Bringing us to a necessary 'crisis' in the root sense of the word – a decisive 'turning point' in our lives.

- Allowing us to fully express and reveal intense emotional pain by feeling and expressing it as a reaction to physical pain.

- Incapacitating us in a way that allows us to accept real limits to our capacities – limits we might otherwise have sought (or been put under pressure) to deny and overcome.

- Letting us become dependent on others in a socially acceptable way, and in this way to express dependency needs which we might otherwise think are unacceptable.

- Enabling us to indirectly ask for and receive emotional care and attention from others through the care of our bodies and being taken care of as 'patients'.

- Helping us to give more time and be more patient with ourselves and others by becoming 'a patient'.

- Providing a temporary respite from life problems by becoming a medical 'patient' in need of treatment and care.

- Providing a temporary but coherent organising principle for a person's life – built around their symptoms or around timetables of rest and treatment.

- Overcoming isolation and offering a medium of human contact through relationships with physicians or through the social environment of a hospital ward.

- Putting us into an altered state of consciousness – one in which we can come to feel ourselves and see our lives in a different way.

- Stopping us from just living in our heads and minds and helping us feel our bodies again – thereby giving us a fuller, more embodied sense of self.

- Transforming our 'body identity' and 'body speech' – bringing about and giving birth to a new bodily sense of who we are and new bodily ways of relating to others.

- Allowing us to identify with and feel close to an important person in our lives – living or deceased – who may have suffered symptoms of illnesses similar to our own.

- Giving symbolic expression to a subjectively felt *dis-ease.* For example heart conditions as a metaphorical expression of either 'loss of heart' or 'heartlessness', 'cold-heartedness' or 'faint-heartedness' etc.

- Giving birth to a new bodily sense of self or 'body identity' – one more in tune with one's current life, able to relate in new ways to others and respond in new ways to one's life world.

Finally, we must not forget the importance of illness as a quite natural way of dying or as a way out of intolerable life circumstances such as extreme poverty or war. The 'war' that biological medicine wages on disease on the other hand, is part of a wholly unnatural and wholly unwinnable war against the basic *life* realities of both aging and *death*. That is why people seek cosmetic or herbal 'elixirs' of youth and science seeks to develop bio-technologies that offer a purely physical form of immortality. What this reveals is a social culture that values quantitative longevity over quality of life, and why biomedicine uses all possible means – even the most toxic – to extend the lives of patients by mere months – at whatever economic cost and at whatever cost to a patient's *quality of life.*

Basic Guides to Self-Healing

1. Meditating Specific Symptoms

- Give yourself time to be aware of your immediate *bodily* sensations of any state of illness or dis-ease. Ask yourself and become more aware *of where and how* you feel your dis-ease in your body.

- Remind yourself that the pure awareness of any sensation, emotion or thought – however painful – is *not itself* a sensation, emotion or thought, and is innately pain free.

- Staying aware of any localised sensation or symptom, remind yourself that it is itself *an awareness* of some aspect of your life-world and relationships that is a source of unease or 'dis-ease'.

- Wait until a spontaneous awareness arises of what specific aspect of your life-world it is that the sensation or feeling of dis-ease embodies – and is itself an awareness *of*.

- Grant awareness to one localised sensation or feeling of dis-ease or discomfort after another, staying with it long enough until it too recalls you to some specific aspect of your life world, present, past or future.

- Take time to follow this process through – making sure you attend to every region of your body *in* the process – until your *overall* sense of dis-ease lifts and your overall sense of self and body alters – transformed by the very awareness you are granting it.

2. Cultivating Whole-Body Awareness of Dis-ease

- Remember: only through awareness of your *body as a whole* can you gain and maintain a sense of your *self as a whole* – your 'soul'.

- When you feel ill therefore, do not focus solely on your symptoms – on localised sensations, thoughts or emotions – but instead seek to maintain a sense of your body, self and life *as whole*.

- If you feel yourself suffering from what you think of as a purely 'mental' or emotional state, remember that every such state is always accompanied by a particular *bodily* sense of yourself.

- Conversely therefore, even if your symptoms seem to be purely bodily, attend also to the thoughts and emotions that tend to accompany them – for these will give you the best clue to the underlying life-problem that they symbolise.

- Understand too, that any mental, emotional and bodily state that you experience when you feel ill is at the same time a 'self state' or 'body identity' – a particular bodily way of feeling *yourself* – who you are.

- Attend therefore, not only to the way your symptoms 'make you feel' but to the way they make *you* feel – the overall sense of self or 'body identity' that accompanies them.

- If you can, *choose* to fully feel and indeed even amplify any felt sensations of dis-ease or sickness symptoms rather than seeking to suppress them.

- *Trust* that any mood or feeling, sense of dis-ease or bodily symptom – if it is given *enough time* to be fully felt, amplified and inwardly followed – will in time *automatically transform* itself into a new feeling, a new sense of your body and a new bodily sense of self or 'body identity' – one now free of the need to embody or 'somatise' itself through symptoms of one sort or another.

Note:

The lack of whole-body awareness *as such* in our generally mind and head-oriented culture is itself a type of basic social pathology – one that is not resolved through simply placing equal emphasis on the heart and emotions as well as on the head and intellect. For both thoughts and emotions are experienced in localised ways and in localised regions of the body. Authentic whole-body awareness on the other hand, is comparable to the awareness of one's body as whole – from top to toe, inside and outside – that is experienced in the womb, and that also arises when, for example, one enters and comes to rest in a hot bath. Maintaining whole body awareness means that this sensation of warmth pervading one's whole body – and maintaining one's awareness of it - persists unbroken, through out the day. Put in other words the body as a whole – though having long left the warm and fluid waters of the womb – is itself experienced as a safe, fluid and warmth-filled womb of the self.

Illness as an Awareness

Every feeling, symptom, mental or physical state, together with our overall sense of self or 'self-state' is not just something we are aware *of*. Its meaning lies in the fact that *it is itself an awareness* of something. Thus a muscular tension, for example in the form of a tension headache, though we only be aware of it as a bodily tension, may itself embody an awareness of a particular tension in our lives, relationships or place of work.

Just as a person whose family has been made homeless or wiped out in a war has *good reasons* for feeling 'sick' or 'depressed', so do all feelings and symptoms have good reasons. They are not just programmed or mechanical physiological reactions to or 'effects' of external or internal 'causes'. Simply to label feelings as 'positive' or 'negative', to describe ourselves as 'well' or 'unwell', or to call the way we feel as 'good' or 'bad', is to deny the inherent *meaning* of all feelings – as an awareness of something beyond themselves. Symptoms of illness, like dream symbols, are a form of *condensed* awareness. Their *inherently* positive value and meaning lies in helping us to become more *directly* aware of what it is that they themselves *are* a condensed or embodied awareness of. Thus digestive problems are a condensed embodied awareness of an aspect of our lives or lived experience of the world we find difficult to 'stomach' or 'digest'.

Even though illness is often or mainly experienced through *localised* bodily symptoms (including 'mental' states such as a sense of confusion localised in our heads), every such symptom is also and always accompanied by a state of consciousness or 'mood' that pervades *our entire body* and in this way also affects our entire *bodily sense of self*. This bodily sense of self or 'self-state' is itself an undifferentiated *awareness* of what may be many different aspects of our overall *life world* that are difficult or uncomfortable, distressing or disturbing for us – thus giving rise to a general sense of 'dis-ease'. That is why, in order to find meaning in the overall bodily sense of 'unwellness' or 'dis-ease' that accompanies a specific illness, it is necessary first to experience it *as* a self-state. This means giving awareness to how any state of discomfort or dis-ease, however localised, imparts a specific overall tone, texture and colour to our subjectively felt body or 'lived body' *as a whole* – in this way lending also a specific tone and colour to our bodily sense of self or 'body identity' and to our experienced or lived *world* as a whole.

To pass from an experience of illness as 'not feeling ourselves' to one of 'feeling another self' – a distinct self or 'self-state' – means experiencing this distinct bodily sense of self. The 'other self' we experience through illness however is, by definition, *an experienced self* – a self we are aware *of*. Our self as a whole or 'soul' on the other hand, is not essentially any *experienced* self, symptom, state of consciousness or 'self-state', but rather the very *awareness* of experiencing it. To avoid becoming unconsciously identified with the self-states and symptoms of dis-ease, it is necessary to identify with that 'whole self' which is nothing *but* this awareness – the *experiencing self* rather than any *experienced self*. Only within the awareness that *is* this self – our 'awareness self' – can we in turn feel and affirm every particular feeling and self we experience or are aware *of*. We are as much aware of our *self as a whole* – our soul – as we are aware of our *body* as a whole. Yet the 'body' of our whole self or soul – our *awareness self* – is not just our physical body but *our entire life world*. For it is an awareness that embraces everything and 'every-body' in our world, from our immediate present reality and relationships to our past and future – and ultimately the entire universe.

The *second* step in healing ourselves through awareness is therefore to experience each and every localised bodily sensation or symptom, no matter how subtle, *as an awareness* of some specific aspect of our larger body – of our life world. Thus by giving more awareness to a localised muscular tension we can experience it *as* an awareness of a specific tension in our life world. Through a meditational process of giving awareness to each and every *localised* bodily feeling or sensation of dis-ease – no matter how subtle, and by making sure we attend to each and every *region* of our body in the process – we can come to experience each of these feelings and sensations *as* an awareness of some aspect of our larger body or life world. Through this process we are literally putting ourselves together – 're-membering' and making whole that larger body that is our life world *as a whole*. By simply *granting* awareness to each region of our bodies and each sensation or feeling of dis-ease or discomfort we experience within it, our overall sense of dis-ease and overall 'self-state' will automatically begin to alter. For we will feel ever-more pervaded, lightened and healed by that very self which is the *awareness* we grant to our overall self-state – our body, self and our life world *as a whole*.

Case Example 2
Two Ways of Responding to Symptoms

1. A personal secretary finds herself stuck in a job with a bullying and abusive boss. Fearing to express her feelings of irritation, anger and humiliation 'face to face' and 'face up to' her boss, feeling vulnerable in the face of the unpredictable rage this might unleash in her boss, and afraid with good reason that it might be 'rash' to risk her job by doing so, she keeps 'a straight face' in the face of all the bullying. Over time her feelings come to the surface in her body itself – in the form of an 'irritating' and 'angry' red skin rash. Lacking a way to 'face up to' her boss, let alone 'whack him one' – even though she is itching to do so – the rash appears on her face, arms and hands. Plagued by itching, she scratches and irritates her own skin until it blisters and bleeds – an activity that provides, unaware to herself, some satisfaction in releasing her 'bad blood' towards her boss. But her feelings of embarrassment and shame about not being able to face up to her boss become displaced by shame and embarrassment about the rash itself. So she goes to her doctor. Not even thinking that asking her questions about her life world might have any diagnostic significance, the doctor is therefore completely blind to the metaphorical *meaning* of her 'angry rash'. Adopting a conventional medical approach, the doctor's sole interest is in diagnosing the rash as some form of skin disorder and treating it – and prescribes a cortisone cream. The problem is that she then becomes dependent on the cream, which far from helping her to become tougher and more 'thick-skinned' emotionally, has the side-effect of thinning her actual skin surface itself, making it more vulnerable to embarrassing sores and bleeding. Eventually she feels forced to either lash out at her boss and risk being fired or else to leave her job voluntarily and seek another boss.

2. The same secretary allows herself to fully feel the emotions of anger, vulnerability, shame and humiliation she experiences. This means allowing herself to feel them fully in her body as a whole, neither repressing them nor being provoked to *rashly* reacting from them. She allows herself to *be* angry rather than 'getting angry'. She also reminds herself that the pure awareness of an emotion, however intense, is not itself an emotion or impulse but something innately emotion- and impulse-free. Letting herself *feel* and *be* angry makes her feel less vulnerable to her boss's bullying. Instead the anger transforms itself into an awareness of the bullying that allows her to see it for what it really is – as the expression of a deep insecurity and vulnerability in her boss himself. At the same time, by bearing her anger and feeling it fully in her body, it transforms into a sense of a different self within her, a self strong enough to face up to her boss – or to anyone – in a calm, non-hostile but nevertheless firm and resolute way. By *bodying* this new self through her body language and tone of voice she feels ever less vulnerable to her boss and instead becomes aware of the vulnerability behind his bullying. Sensing this, he finds it strangely more difficult to be as bullying towards her as before. For now it is *he* who is aware of feeling an insecure, vulnerable self behind his anger. Initially fearing this self, he first intensifies his abusive bullying, only to find it met by a calm, resolute and firmly toned response from the secretary. Not being able to provoke her into 'getting angry' the secretary is not fired. And being now capable of bodying her anger through a new inner bearing she no longer needs to 'somatise' it through an angry red facial rash, or fear being fired.

Illness as an Altered State of Consciousness

From the point of view of Life Medicine there is no need to scientifically find or prove causal links or relations between 'body and mind', 'body and brain'. Instead it is a matter of recognising that every bodily state *is* a 'mental' state, but in a much broader sense than usually understood – being a state of consciousness that is experienced just as much in a bodily way as in our 'minds'.

No 'subjective' state or 'state of consciousness' is merely something enclosed or encapsulated in our heads, brains or minds. Conversely the body as such is not something we merely perceive or are merely aware of 'mentally' – as if it were some object we carry around with us. Instead the body itself is but a particular shape and dimension of subjective experiencing – one that completely transcends the whole body-mind, body-brain division. This is why the notion of the 'felt body', 'lived body' or 'subjective body' is so central to Life Medicine – and to the new understanding of illness it brings. For this new understanding makes it impossible, in principle, to separate our lived experience of illness into two separate categories that we call 'mental' and 'physical'.

A basic principle of Life Medicine is that every *bodily state* is also a *state of consciousness* and vice versa. That is why the experience of any bodily state or condition, even a minor ailment such as a flu or cold goes together with a new and different state of consciousness – a state of consciousness that is not limited to one's head or mind but pervades one's entire body.

Conversely, different types of 'mental' or 'emotional' states are also states of consciousness not confined to the head or mind – but felt and experienced in a bodily way, for example as a particular sensation arising from a state of muscular tension in one's chest, stomach or guts.

"Every feeling is... a mood that embodies in this or that way."

Martin Heidegger

What we call a 'mood' however, is nothing we are simply mentally aware of in our heads, but is rather a particular tone and quality of embodied, feeling awareness – one which is always in one way embodied as different degrees and qualities of *muscle tone and tension* – which is why no state of 'mental' stress or tension is not at the same time a state of muscular tension.

"A mood makes manifest how one is..." Martin Heidegger

In other words, a mood is not just something purely mental but is a bodily way of *feeling ourselves*. This is reflected in the fact that the question *'How do you feel?'* is synonymous with the *question 'How are you?'* For the way we 'feel' is the way we 'are' – and vice versa.

For this reason however, any alteration or change in *how* we feel or are is at the same time a change in our sense of *who* we are or feel ourselves to be – a change in our identity or sense of self that is felt in an immediate bodily way. For in a most literal sense the 'you' that feels sick or tired is not the *same* 'you' that feels healthy, bright and alert.

Thus, not only is every *bodily state* also a *state of consciousness* – it could also be described as a 'self-state' or 'body identity'. For the way we feel our bodies cannot be separated from the way we feel ourselves. *How* we feel in our body affects not just our mind but *who* we feel ourselves to be – our 'bodily sense of self' or 'body identity'. That is why, when people begin to feel ill they might speak of 'not feeling themselves'. This basic 'dis-ease' of 'not feeling ourselves' is both the essence and first sign of illness – being not only an altered state of consciousness (how we feel) but also an alteration of our bodily sense of self or body identity – of *who* we feel ourselves to be.

The Immune System and Body Identity

In the framework of biomedicine 'body identity' is reduced to our genetic or *biological* identity and associated in particular with the immune system - which is seen as 'defending' our biological identity against threats and attacks from 'foreign bodies' in the form of pathogenic bacteria, viruses or mutant and cancerous cells, or any type of genetic material such as organ transplants that consist of 'non-self' cells (a term actually used in immunology).

Today more than ever, much fuss is made about 'health' being dependent on maintaining or restoring a strong 'immune system' or with strengthening the body's immune 'defences', which is why countless food products and supplements are advertised that claim to do so. On the other hand even biomedicine acknowledges that most discomforting or painful symptoms of illness (such as a runny nose or swelling and painful joints) arise from the activity of the body's immune system. Indeed many illnesses are recognised as resulting from an immune system that is too strongly defensive and as a result is *overactive* - leading to so-called 'autoimmune' diseases such as arthritis in which the body's immune 'defences' are used to attack its own cells. Alternatively, the body's immune system may be at such a high alert and so overactive and 'strong' for long periods that it ultimately weakens or collapses. Its very strength and activity therefore may ultimately result in precisely the sort of weakness that makes the body susceptible to infection and other types of illness.

In contrast to biomedicine, Life Medicine understands the strength of our immune system – the degree of immunity of our *bodies* – as an *embodiment* of the degree of immunity of our *self* or *identity*. Thus a *too rigid* or *strongly defended* identity or sense of self – one completely 'immune' to natural and healthy processes of *change* and adaptation to life - may find biological expression through an *over-defensive* and *over-active* immune system, which then actively seeks out threats to our biological identity that would otherwise be ignored or are ignored by the immune systems of other people. An over-rigid or immune *self* – or one that experiences deep *identity conflicts* - would explain many so-called 'auto-immune' disorders. A more healthily and naturally 'strong' identity or sense of self on the other hand would also explain what biomedical immunology can't explain – why some people 'catch' diseases which are supposed to be highly infectious whilst others don't – even from spouses or children they live with or during widespread epidemics. Nor can biomedical immunology explain why most of the bacteria, viruses and even damaged, mutated and 'cancerous' cells that biological medicine regards as 'causes' of diseases are all in fact *constantly present* in most healthy bodies.

Biomedicine simply takes it for granted that 'health' is the protection of a *fixed* biological and genetic identity – one 'immune' from all change. The problem with this theory is that it prevents biomedicine from coming up with any explanation of why it is that the immune system, though it may launch attacks on transplanted cells and tumours, does *not* launch attacks on a no less alien or foreign body that can grow within the human body – namely the baby growing in a pregnant mother's womb? And whilst biomedicine has effectively come to treat pregnancy and birth as something fraught with as many dangers as an illness, therefore requiring hospitalisation and the use of hi-tech medical equipment, the body itself clearly does not regard pregnancy as a disease or the baby as an alien or foreign body growing inside it – despite the differences in its DNA to that of the mother. Life Medicine, on the other hand, understands 'health' itself as a capacity to allow our body identity or sense of self to be altered and transformed in response to our life world and life experiences. That is why, instead of *treating pregnancy as if it were a type of illness*, Life Medicine understands *illness itself as a type of pregnancy* – the meaning and purpose of which is precisely to allow us to gestate and give birth to a new 'bodily sense of self' or 'body identity'. A key aspect of health, not as a mere state but as an on-going *life process* is therefore the capacity to pass from a state of 'not feeling ourselves' to one of 'feeling another self' – and of learning to embody or 'give birth' to that self through new and different ways of relating to our lives and life world.

Health and Illness as Life Processes

The different ways in which it is possible to interpret and respond to discomforting alterations in our bodily sense of self – in particular that bodily sense of 'not feeling ourselves' that accompanies even the most *minor* of symptoms such as feeling a cold or flu coming on – take us to the very heart of the contrast between Biomedicine and Life Medicine. They also enable us to understand both health and illness as self-states and *life processes* rather than merely as bodily states or biological processes.

A key aspect of both health *and* illness as *life processes* is how we interpret and respond to the essential 'dis-ease' of 'not feeling ourselves' – a dis-ease that may either precede or accompany discomforting symptoms of illness. One option is to feel this dis-ease and its symptoms merely as a *sign* of some biological disease or disorder – leading to what I call 'the illness process'. An alternative is to feel our dis-ease as a state or pregnancy and our bodily state as the womb of a new and different sense of self gestating within us – a self we do not need to 'defend' against or 'fight' with our body's immune system. This is what I call 'the health process' in contrast to 'the illness process', the stages of both of which are described below:

The Health Process

1. 'Feeling ourselves' in a familiar and 'normal' way that we identify with feeling 'healthy'.

2. 'Not feeling ourselves' – feeling a change in our bodily sense of self or body identity.

3. Choosing to actively affirm and identify with our altered bodily sense of self or 'body identity'.

4. Giving ourselves time to meditate our felt-disease in the context of our current lives.

5. Passing from 'not feeling ourselves' to 'feeling another self' – to experiencing the change in our bodily sense of self not as something that is 'not me' or 'other than self' but as a distinct self in its own right.

6. Seeking to actively embody and in this way give birth to the new sense of self that is pregnant in our dis-ease through new ways of being and relating to others and our life world.

The Illness Process

1. 'Feeling ourselves' in a familiar and 'normal' way that we identify with feeling 'healthy'.

2. 'Not feeling ourselves' – and experiencing this both as a felt sense of *dis-ease* and as the result of some 'thing' that is 'not self' or 'other than self'.

3. Identifying our felt dis-ease solely with some purely bodily state or illness symptom.

4. Seeing this symptom only as a sign of some 'thing' that is 'wrong' with us – such as a medically recognised 'disease'.

5. Seeking a medical diagnosis or 'cause' for our symptoms in some 'foreign body' such as a virus.

6. Seeking a 'cure' for our symptoms by some means of medically counteracting or cutting out that 'foreign body'.

The illness process is always culturally and linguistically shaped. Thus, whilst modern medicine might seek the cause of disease in a foreign body such as a 'malignant' tumour or 'pathogenic' virus or bacterium, a witch-doctor or shaman might blame it on a malign spirit just as earliest Greek physicians blamed illnesses on 'ill-winds' or *pneuma.* Yet what *all* historical forms of medicine have tended to share in common is that any sense of 'not feeling ourselves' – rather than being taken as an opportunity to begin 'feeling another self' – is instead identified with feeling something wholly 'other than self' such as a foreign body or spirit, or a 'non-self' cell or organism. In this way however, the health process – passing from 'not feeling ourselves' to 'feeling another self' is *foreclosed* and gives way instead to the 'illness process'.

Illness as Pregnancy and the Life Doctor as Midwife

If we understand illness in the framework of Life Medicine, i.e. as a life process comparable to gestation, then all forms of medical treatment or 'cure' are equivalent to an attempt to medically 'terminate' or 'abort' the new bodily sense of self or 'body identity' that is pregnant in the patient's dis-ease. Such premature medical termination or abortion of an illness has the immediate 'side effect' of preventing the patient from taking time to explore, understand and identify more clearly the new sense of self they are gestating and pregnant with – and to find ways of giving birth to it through a new way of living and relating. Abortive biomedical treatment may and does also frequently 'miscarry' in several others ways – not just through other side effects but also through actually intensifying the 'illness process' – the process by which a felt dis-ease is 'somatised' and as a result may take the form of ever more chronic or acute medical symptoms and diseases. Finally, even if a disease or its symptoms *are* cured – whether through conventional medicine, alternative medicine or 'spiritual' healing - if the underlying dis-ease behind it is not explored, the result may well be that the patient simply gives expression to this dis-ease through *other* symptoms or *another* disease - one that may be worse or more serious than the one supposedly 'cured'.

The 'health process' is a process of giving ourselves time to feel ourselves more deeply into a felt dis-ease with the aim of sensing it as an expression of a different bodily sense of self – rather than simply seeking to counteract or cure, suppress or exorcise its symptoms. Since so few people are able to approach any felt sense of dis-ease in this way however – through 'the health process' – this dis-ease may need to take the form of ever more acute or chronic disease symptoms for them to begin to do so. The illness process therefore, can also provide a spur for the health process. Yet if, through the illness process, an individual's *dis-ease* has already reached the point of transforming itself into a serious biological disease, then some form of biomedical intervention may be unavoidable, if only to alleviate its symptoms.

This is precisely the point at which Life Doctoring becomes so vital and relevant - even if conducted in parallel with medical doctoring. For only Life Doctoring can ensure a true 'healing process' is set into train. Here the role of the Life Doctor is to serve as *midwife* for the patient – helping them to give birth to changes in their sense of self or body identity and not just their body, and to changes in their life as a whole and not just their bodily life.

Life Doctoring sessions serve to support this healing and birthing process by offering times and ways for the patient to step back from purely biomedical diagnoses, prognoses and treatments of their illness and by helping them both feel into and come to understand the deeper meaning and purpose of their illness – thus restoring the health process in place of the illness process. The Life Doctor can also play a vital role in helping the patient to consider more carefully and if necessary reject potentially dangerous or high-risk forms of diagnostic testing, treatment or surgery.

For the danger is that these may either miscarry, worsen the patient's symptoms or hasten the progression of their disease – and in any one of these ways result in their premature death. On the other hand, even if medical treatments for serious or terminal diseases *are* 'successful' in purely biomedical terms, they may massively reduce the patient's *quality of life* – merely to extend that life for what is often only a very minimal period.

The Focus of Life Medicine –
The Lived Body

"It is the great error of Western philosophers that they always regard the human body intellectually, from the outside, as though it were not indissolubly a part of the active self."

Sato Tsuji

Which body is it with which we feel ourselves – our self?

Which body is it through which we feel ourselves inwardly 'closer' or more 'distant' to others, however near or far they are in physical space and time?

Which body is it with which we can feel ourselves to be inwardly 'warmer' or 'cooler' towards other people, irrespective of our physical temperature?

Which body is it with which we can feel ourselves inwardly as 'heavier' or 'lighter', 'fatter' or 'thinner', yet without any change to our physical weight or size?

Which body is it whose 'heart' can be inwardly felt as 'big' or 'small', 'warm' or 'cold', with which we or others can feel 'heartened' or 'disheartened', 'lose heart' or suffer 'heartache', seem 'heartless' or 'big hearted' - independently of the size or functioning of 'the heart' as a physical organ?

Which body is it with which we can feel ourselves 'expanding' or 'shrinking', 'uplifted' or 'carried away', 'sucked in' or 'trapped', 'open' or 'closed off', 'full' or 'empty', 'shapeless' or 'spineless', 'exploding' or 'imploding' – yet without our physical body moving or changing shape in any way?

Which body is it with which we can feel inwardly 'drawn into', 'drawn out of' – or 'withdrawn into' ourselves – as if into some warm and nurturing womb or else some cold and solitary prison or tomb?

Which body is it with which we feel 'high' or 'low', 'up' or 'down', 'uplifted' or 'let down', 'beside ourselves', 'spaced out' or confined in our skins?

Which body is it whose 'skin' we feel more or less inwardly 'at home' in, which can make someone seem 'thick- or thin-skinned', that without any physical skin irritations can make us feel 'prickly', 'edgy' or 'irritable', 'stretched' or 'frayed', that can feel tight and constricting like a diving suit or straightjacket – or like a porous, comfortable and loose-fitting garment?

Which body is it that can be felt as more or less inwardly 'solid' or 'firm', 'fluid' or 'airy', 'hard' or 'soft', 'smooth' and 'rounded' or 'jagged' and 'sharp edged' – all independently of its physical shape and features?

Which body is it with which we feel the inner 'brightness' or 'darkness', 'levity' or 'gravity', 'lightness' or 'heaviness' of our own and other peoples' moods?

Which body is it whose overall mood or 'feeling tone' – like its voice tone – can be felt as 'bright or dark', 'light or heavy', 'sharp' or 'dull' and 'flat', 'resonant' and 'full' or 'hollow' and 'empty'?

Which body is it that we actually sense and feel from within, that is the source of all bodily proprioception and self-experiencing – rather than a mere object of perception for others?

The answer to all these questions is not our fleshly 'physical' body and its organs. It is not any body we can measure or weigh.

Nor, however, is it some form of pseudo-physical 'energy body' of the sort that New Agers and practitioners of alternative medicine speak of (see *Life Medicine and 'Energy Medicine'*).

Instead it is our 'felt body' or 'lived body' – the body of our feeling *awareness* of ourselves, other people and our life world as a whole.

The lived body is not composed of tissue, bone and blood, cells and organs, but of the 'stuff' that Shakespeare spoke of – that "stuff on which dreams are made".

The lived body is therefore also the body as we experience it in our dreams – what Arnold Mindell calls the 'dreambody' or 'dreaming body'. And yet it is also more, being the very 'life and soul' of our physical body.

For what I term *feeling awareness* is what *used* to be called the 'soul' or 'psyche' – yet in a way that traditionally has failed to recognise the 'soul' or 'psyche' *as* a body in its own right – the lived body as a body *of* feeling awareness.

It is the lived body or 'soul body' that quite literally 'in-forms' the flesh or 'physical' body. And yet it is in no way bounded by our skin in the way that our physical body is.

For, as the body of our subjective, feeling awareness of ourselves the lived body (German *Leib*) embraces all that we feel and experience in our life, not just through the physical body and in the entire life world that surrounds it.

The physical body on the other hand, is but one part of that larger life world as a whole and thus also just one outward expression and embodiment of our lived body as a whole.

So the terms 'lived body' or 'felt body' should not be thought of as referring simply to the 'physical body' as we feel or experience it from within. Instead it is the other way round. What we call the 'physical body' is nothing but the lived body as it appears to us and others "from the outside".

That is why no form of 'objective' external or even 'internal' examination or scanning of the physical body – which just means viewing the inside of the physical body "from the outside" – will ever reveal the lived body - which is a distinct *subjective body* in its own right.

The lived body is not made up of molecules, cells, tissue and organs but of patterned tones, textures and flows of feeling awareness - including molecular, cellular and organic awareness. It is these *organising* patterns and textures of mood or 'feeling tone' which not only shape and compose our awareness but also shape and pervade our lived body *as* an 'organism'.

Of course, it is difficult to persuade a 'scientific' biologist that behind what appears "from the outside" as a mere 3-dimensional physical object in the form of the physical body or 'organism' lies a body – the lived body – made up of organising patterns and tones of feeling awareness. For these are invisible to any microscope and undetectable by any scanning devices.

That is also why trying to persuade medical scientists and practitioners of 'the lived body' is like trying to persuade *people who have not learned to read* that behind the 3-dimensional form of a book, the chemical ink marks on its 2-dimensional pages or the electronic pixels on a flat screen of text lies an invisible yet multidimensional world of *living meaning* – one which no form of chemical analysis or of radiographical or magnetic scanning can ever reveal. For this is a world that we can only enter and experience, discover and find 'evidence' of by first learning to *read* the book or text.

Yet just as the physical body can be compared to a book or text, so is it also a *speech organ* of the soul and of its body – the lived body. This truth finds expression in body language, in the many bodily 'metaphors' that pervade verbal language itself (such as 'losing heart' or finding something 'hard to 'stomach') as well as in the symptoms of illness itself, understood as bodily symbols.

Body language or 'body speech', bodily metaphors and physical symptoms are at the same time all ways in which the 'physical body' reveals itself as a living 'bio-logical' expression of the *lived body* in a literal sense – being its 'life speech' or *bios logos*. This is what Freud called 'organ speech' (*Organsprache*).

'Organic Disease' as 'Organ Speech'

"Through the long succession of millennia, man has not known himself physiologically; he does not know himself even today."

Friedrich Nietzsche

Do failing organs or disturbances to the functioning of their physiological capacities lead to illness – or are organic or physiological functions and capacities the embodiment of capacities of another sort – capacities of feeling awareness?

Thus when we speak of someone 'losing heart', feeling 'disheartened' or 'heart-broken', for example, we are not just using the language of a biological 'organ' – in this case the heart – as a mere metaphor for a psychological state or sense of 'dis-ease'. It is the other way round. Heart disease is itself *a living biological metaphor* of subjective states of dis-ease and distress such as feeling 'heart-broken', 'heartless' or 'cold-hearted'.

Similarly, respiratory disorders such as asthma arise from a subjective sense of feeling 'stifled' or 'having no room to breathe' in our lives, just as digestive disorders are the expression of aspects of our lived experience and life world that we do not feel able to 'stomach' or 'digest' in our awareness.

Biological medicine seeks 'organic' causes for illness in dysfunctions of our *physiological organs* – and sees even psychological disorders as the result of such organic dysfunctions, as disorders of our brain chemistry. As a result, biological medicine is blind to the deeper meaning and truth of the bodily language and 'metaphors' we use to describe what are usually thought of only as 'mental' or 'psychological' feelings and states. It does not see that the language of these bodily metaphors is a way of recognising that the physical body and its organs are not a biological machine or a mere product of our genes but a *living biological language* of the human being.

In contrast, Freud spoke of bodily symptoms as a type of organic language or 'organ speech' (*Organsprache*). Similarly, Life Medicine recognises all organs and functions of the 'physical' body as the biological expression of organised capacities and functions of another body – our 'lived body' – the body of our feeling awareness of all that we experience in our lives.

In German there are not one but two words for 'the body' – *Körper* and *Leib*. The only equivalents of *Körper* in English are the words 'corpus' and 'corpse'. 'Corpse' is also the root meaning of the Greek word 'soma', from which the term 'somatic' derives. It refers of course to a dead body as opposed to a living one. There is however another German word for body – *Leib* – that can be translated as 'lived body' or 'life' body – for it is part of a whole family of words to do with 'life' (*Leben*) and 'living' (*leben*). These words include *erleben* ('to experience') and *Erlebnis* (an experience). Through the inner lens of the German language in other words, life (*Leben*) and living (*leben*) are understood essentially as realm of *subjective experiencing* (*er-leben*). Thus the body as *Leib* or 'lived body' refers to our own 'experienced' and 'experiencing' body' – the body of our living *experience* of ourselves, our lives and our entire life world. The basic 'capacities' of the lived body or *Leib* therefore have to do with what we are or are not able to do with our experience (*Erlebnis*) of living (*leben*), of life (*Leben*) and of our 'life world' (*Lebenswelt*).

In physiological terms, the capacities of the lived body are our capacity to *sense, perceive, breathe in, digest* and *metabolise* all that we experience, allowing it to *circulate* within our awareness and thus *nourish* our very *being* with life-giving *meaning*.

Both our sense organs and other biological organs such as our lungs, stomach and heart, together with their corresponding physiological functions, are essentially nothing but organic and physiological *embodiments* of capacities belonging to our lived body as a 'psychical organism' or 'body of awareness' – an awareness *more or less* open to or capable of sensuously embracing, feeling and perceiving, breathing in, digesting and metabolising all that we experience in our lives – and in this way extracting meaning from it.

On the other hand, any *lack or dysfunction* of these basic capacities of awareness belonging to the lived body may also *embody* itself – finding expression in what biomedicine then sees only as purely 'physiological' or 'organic' dysfunctions, disorders or 'diseases' – for example respiratory, digestive, metabolic or circulatory diseases.

"We cannot say that the organ has capacities, but must say that the capacity has organs... capability, articulating itself into capacities creating organs characterises the organism as such."

Martin Heidegger

The idea that biological organs are a "creation" or embodiment of the very capabilities or capacities we associate with that organ is of course a revolutionary one.

Yet along with the family of German words that includes the 'lived body' (*Leib*), 'life' (*Leben*) and experiencing (*er-leben*) goes another word that hints at how this idea may be understood: the verb 'to body' (*leiben*).

For as Heidegger remarked in addressing a circle of doctors:

"We know by now a great deal – almost more than we can encompass – about what we call the body, without having seriously thought about what <u>bodying</u> is ... The bodying of life is nothing separate by itself, encapsulated in the 'physical mass' in which the body can appear to us..."

Hence also the profound significance of another insight of his, namely that:

"Every feeling is an embodiment attuned in this or that way, a mood that embodies in this or that way."

It is through the lived body that we quite literally embody or 'body' felt tones or 'moods' of feeling awareness or 'feeling tones' – allowing them to find expression in cellular tone, skin tone, muscle and organ tone, i.e. in 'organ speech' – as well as in the tones of our vocal speech. The lived body then, is the very source and essence of the human 'organism'.

For it is that musical or tonal 'instrument' (the root meaning of the Greek word *organon* from which the term 'organism' is derived) through which we inwardly 'speak' or 'utter' our organs themselves from out of shaped and patterned tones of feeling awareness or 'feeling tones'. For, what are sound, music and speech except a shaping or patterning of tone?

Yet feeling tones can be either healthy and 'sound' or else more or less muddied, discordant and 'unsound'. This is also the reason we speak of someone's health or a particular organ being or not being in 'sound' condition, and associate health with 'soundness', the words *sound* and *soundness* being the root meaning of the German words for 'healthy' and 'health' – *gesund* and *Gesundheit.*

The human organism then – indeed *any* organism – is nothing 'biological' or 'organic' in the narrow scientific sense. It is 'biological' only in the essential sense of being that instrument or *organon* through which 'life' (*bios*) speaks itself in the form of fleshly organs – giving physical shape and tone to felt patterns, shapes, tones and textures of feeling awareness.

The essence of any organism consists of *organising field patterns of awareness*. These in turn are what give ordered and organised shape and form to that larger *patterned field of awareness* that constitutes the perceived 'environment' or *life world* of any organism.

Human *language* too is an organised and organising structure, one which shapes and patterns our specifically human awareness and perception of the world. And language itself is made up of 'organising patterns of awareness' that make it an integral part of the lived body – and not a mere function of something we call 'the mind' or of the brain as a biological organ.

It is because it is an *integral part* of the human organism that the body and its organs itself figure so strongly in *language itself* – in countless everyday expressions relating to bodily *organs* such as the heart (feeling 'disheartened' or 'a stab in the heart), to *parts* of the body ('having one's feet on the ground') and bodily functions such as respiration (feeling 'stifled' or having 'no room to breathe').

The body even figures in the mere use of *simple prepositions* such as 'in' and 'out', 'on' and 'off', 'up' and 'down' – for example being 'onto' or 'into' something', feeling 'up' or 'down', 'high' and 'low', 'off colour' or 'out of' one's mind. For all these expressions arise from and reflect our felt bodily relation to space – as also does the use of words such as 'upset', 'unstable' or 'imbalanced' and expressions such as 'leaning to one side', 'finding one's ground' or 'shifting' one's stance or attitude, posture or position.

This all-pervasive bodily dimension of language itself – and its roots in bodily experiencing – was first explored in depth by Lakoff and Johnson in their book *Metaphors We Live By*. Yet it also lends support to the basic principles of Life Medicine, as well as to Freud's notion of 'organ speech'. This notion is in turn closely associated with what, in his last years, he came to call 'The Second Fundamental Principle of Psychoanalysis'.

This is the principle that 'bodily' states and symptoms were not merely things that emerged 'parallel' with or 'concomitant' to unconscious mental or 'psychic' states. Instead what were previously thought of in psychoanalysis only as "somatic concomitants" of these states were recognised as "the truly psychical" (Freud).

The radical implication of this principle is that the true foundation and focus of psychoanalysis is not 'the interpretation of dreams' or some mysterious entity called 'the unconscious' but *the language of the body* – which finds expression both in our waking life and in our dreams and 'dreaming body' and is the symbolic key to all forms and symptoms of illness.

Yet the significance of Freud's new 'foundational principle of psychoanalysis' has still not been registered by most psychoanalysts or schools of psychoanalysis – and certainly not in medical theory and practice.

Only through the work of the Argentinean psychoanalyst *Luis Chiozza* did psychoanalysis come to both appreciate and apply this principle.

He did so by recognising, as Life Medicine does, that the two *distinct but inseparable* dimensions of what Freud called 'organ speech' – verbal expression such as 'feeling stifled' or 'stabbed in the heart' on the one hand, and experienced physical sensations or symptoms such as breathing difficulties or heart pains on the other – share a *common source*. In other words, symptoms of illness itself are not only reflected in language that describes felt states of dis-ease. Instead illness itself *is* a language.

As a psychoanalyst, Chiozza saw the common source of illness and language as 'the unconscious'. In Life Medicine this common source is seen as life itself – as experienced through the lived body.

Yet it was Chiozza who also first began to apply the practice of Life Medicine. Derived from Victor von Weizsäcker and called the 'pathobiographical' method, it involves seeking the 'hidden story' behind a patient's illness by finding links between its biology on the one hand, and the biography or life story of the patient on the other. Such links can above all be sought and found through the *language of illness* and through understanding illness itself *as a language*.

References:
Chiozza, Luis A. *Hidden Affects in Somatic Disorders*
Chiozza, Luis A. *Why Do We Fall Ill? – The Story Hiding in the Body*
Heidegger, Martin, *Zollikon Seminars*
Lakoff and Johnson, *Metaphors We Live By*

The Language of Illness & Illness as a Language

Could it be that the way we use language to talk *about* illness and disease affects our whole understanding of it? Could it be that "the essence of a disease" and "the essence of a word" – of the language with which we describe states of 'dis-ease' – are one and the same?

To begin with it is important to recognise how many phrases used to talk about illness contain words that imply that it is:

- some 'thing' that we 'have', 'catch' or 'get'
- something that is 'wrong' or 'bad'
- something that attacks us
- Something that fails

Examples:
- I *caught* a cold.
- She *has* cancer.
- What's *wrong* with me?
- He's got a *bad* heart.
- My back/head is *killing* me.
- He is suffering from liver *failure.*

Secondly, biological medicine, far from being based purely on scientific fact, is pervaded by verbal metaphors or figures of speech - and in particular expressions derived from the language of war and violence.

Examples:

- *War* on cancer.
- *Defending or protecting oneself against* disease.
- *Battling, struggling or fighting against* an illness.
- *Mobilising/reinforcing* the body's immune *defences.*
- An *aggressive* tumour or virus.
- *Fighting off* an infection.
- *Killer* cells.

Thirdly, illness has been explained and interpreted historically in many different religious, moral and 'scientific' ways.

Examples:

- As a punishment for sin.
- As a 'test' of will or faith.
- As an attack by malign spirits.
- As a result of misdeeds in a past life.
- As a sign of moral 'degeneracy' (syphilis, AIDS).
- As an evolutionary means for the survival of the fittest.
- As an invasion by pathogens such as bacteria or viruses.
- As the 'price' paid for an 'unhealthy' lifestyle.
- As a result of eating the 'wrong' foods.
- As a colonisation by cancerous cells.
- As a result of faulty genes.

Fourthly, the body itself has been culturally and linguistically described in many different ways:

Examples:

- As an image of God.
- As a sacred temple of the gods.
- As something to be controlled or tamed by the mind.
- As a container of emotions and of the soul or psyche.
- As a mere disposable shell of the soul or spirit.
- As a more or less well-functioning machine.
- As a product of our genes.

Body Language in Everyday Speech

Everyday speech and verbal language is itself full of 'body language' – containing countless metaphors or 'figures of speech' which not only refer to bodily organs and functions but offer symbolic clues to types of inner dis-ease that might find expression in both physical and mental health problems.

Examples:

- To be/feel *inflamed*, to be *thick-skinned* or *thin-skinned*, *sensitive* or *prickly*, *irritable* or *itchy*, to be *touched* or *untouched* by something/someone, to let something/someone *get under one's skin*.

- To be *heartless* or *cold-hearted*, to *take something to heart*, to be *disheartened*, to *lack heart* or *lose heart*, to be *heartbroken*, a *heartfelt* emotion, a *fluttering heart* etc.

- To find something hard to *stomach* or *digest*, to feel *sick* or *nauseated* about something, to have a *gut feeling* about something, to feel *gutted*.

- To not feel one can *breathe freely*, to feel *stifled*, to feel one has *no room to breathe*, to lack *breathing space*, to lack *inspiration* (from the Latin *spirare* – to breathe).

- To be *headstrong*, to be *boneheaded*, to keep *a clear head*, to *head* in a certain direction, to make or not to make *headway*, to *head something off*, to *have a head* for something, to *lose one's head*, to *bring something to a head* etc.

- To be unable to *face* or *face up* to something or someone, to come *face to face* with something or someone, to *show one's true face*.

- To not *see* a point, to refuse to *see* something, to not *see straight*, to not *see* things in perspective, to lack *vision* or *insight*, to be *short-sighted*, to *close one's eyes* to something, to have a *blindspot*, to not have an *eye* for something.

- To stand on one's own *two feet*, to find one's *balance* or *ground*, to *stand up* for oneself, to take things *in one's stride*.

- To lack *backbone*, to be *spineless*, to *back* someone up or to be in need of support and *backing*.

- To feel inwardly *frozen stiff* or *immobilised*.

- To *shoulder* a burden or lean on someone's shoulders.

- To feel something as a *pain in the neck* or a *pain in the ass*.

- To feel *overstretched, stressed, stiff, constricted* or *tense*.

- To feel someone *getting up one's nose*.

- To be unable to *handle* or *get a grip* on a situation or person.

- To be full of bile.

Even simple linguistic prepositions such as 'in' and 'out', 'on' and 'off', 'up' and 'down' etc – all of which form part and parcel of the very structure of language, play a particularly significant role here, implying that the body is a container of some sort for mental and emotional objects.

Examples:

letting something 'out', taking or holding something 'in', having an idea 'in' one's mind or a feeling 'in' one's body, letting 'out' an emotion, feeling 'off' or 'put off', going 'into' oneself or letting things 'out of' oneself, feeling 'up' or 'down', 'high' or 'low', trapped 'in' one's body or 'out of' one's mind.

All these expressions arise from and reflect our felt bodily relation to space – as also does the use of words such as *'upset', 'unstable' or 'imbalanced'* and expressions such as *'leaning to one side', 'finding one's ground'* or *'shifting' one's stance, attitude, posture or position.*

That language itself *is* 'body language' can also be seen from the way in which expressions referring to 'mental' states make use of figures of speech but relating to specific bodily sensations or movements:

Examples:

feeling 'overstretched' or 'under pressure', 'reaching' for a goal, 'catching' or 'catching onto' something, 'running away' from something', 'moving on' and 'getting ahead', 'falling behind' or 'going downhill', 'falling apart' or putting oneself 'together', 'shaking' with

fear or 'shaking' something off, 'shifting' one's attitude, 'carrying' a
heavy burden, 'grasping', 'hanging onto', 'losing one's grip on' or
'letting go' of something etc.

These are examples of a whole range of expressions used to refer to 'mental' states which at the same time refer to *muscular* states. For example we speak of feeling *tense* or *relaxed*, or else *nervous* or *restless* – hence wanting to fidget or make use of our muscles in some way.

Similarly, a state of high tension or anxiety may be felt muscularly – for example as a 'tension headache', a 'knot' in the stomach, a 'flutter' in the heart etc. This is not surprising given that our heart, stomach and intestines are made up of *muscle* - as are our respiratory and vocal organs.

If someone is drunk or drugged is it their mind or their muscles that may make them feel disoriented or lose their balance? Perhaps it is both and neither. Perhaps it is a person's overall or underlying bodily mood or *tone of feeling* which finds expression both in *muscle tone* and in *mental states*.

Hence also the expression 'highly strung' – which can apply to both a person's nerves and their muscles, but is drawn from the language of stringed musical instruments – and suggests an understanding of the human body or 'organism' itself as a musical instrument – the meaning of the Greek word *organon.*

Finally, both our language and our muscles and joints can be more or less rigid and stiff or *articulate* – allowing us to freely communicate or 'articulate' ourselves through both verbal speech, different tones of voice and 'body speech'. Could it be then, that both illness and language, bodily symptoms and bodily figures of speech

– what Foucault called "the essence of a disease" and the "essence of a word" – are one and the same? Could it be that illness gives this common essence the form of symptoms, whilst language gives it the form of bodily metaphors or figures of speech? Could it be that the body itself is a not a biological machine to be repaired but a *living language* of the human being? For verbal language, as we have seen, is itself largely 'body language' – made up of figures of speech rooted in bodily sensations and states.

Getting to the Heart of Illness –
and of Heart Disease

Listed on the next page is an extended set of everyday expressions, many of which are mentioned in other sections of this book and all of which refer to the 'heart'. Together they 'get to the heart' of what I call the 'felt body' or 'lived body'. For the 'heart' they refer to is not a mere biological organ which mechanically pumps blood, and neither do the expressions refer merely to 'states of mind' separate from and independent of the body. Instead the 'heart' they all refer to is an organ of our lived body rather than our 'physical body'. It is the heart experienced not as a biological organ but as an organ of the lived body – *an organ of feeling awareness.*

"The Language of the Heart"

'a loving heart'

'a passionate heart'

a 'big heart' / a 'kind heart'

a 'cold heart' / 'cold-hearted'

a 'warm heart' / 'warm-hearted'

to be 'open hearted' or 'closed-hearted'

to be 'heart-broken' or 'broken-hearted'

to 'go to' or 'get to' the heart of something'

to be 'hard-hearted' or to 'harden one's heart'

to have or not have the 'heart' for something

to suffer an 'aching heart' or 'heartache'

to be 'heartened' or 'disheartened'

to 'lose heart' or to 'lack heart'

to have a 'heart-to-heart' talk

to feel 'stabbed in the heart'

to 'take something to heart'

to 'strengthen one's heart'

to speak 'from the heart'

to feel one's heart 'sink'

a 'heartfelt emotion'

to be 'heartless'

a 'frozen heart'

'At the heart' of Life Medicine lie three basic understandings all linking Language, Life and Illness:

1. That everyday language referring to *any* of the parts, organs or functions of the human body does not merely make use of bodily 'metaphors' to describe mental or emotional states, but instead indicates the way we live and experience such states in a bodily way – through our subjectively felt body or 'lived body'.

2. That *both* bodily expressions such as 'losing heart' *and* bodily conditions such as heart disease and its symptoms are *symbols* of something else – states and experiences of the felt or lived body and of *its* organs and functions.

3. That so-called 'organic' dysfunctions, disorders or diseases – for example heart diseases – are biological embodiments of basic dysfunctions, disorders or diseases of the lived or felt body: for example an incapacity to feel or love expressed through a hardened heart, or the felt experience of a 'broken heart' or 'loss of heart'.

Life Medicine therefore, does *not* claim that illness is 'all in the mind'. On the contrary, it understands illness – like the many everyday expressions that symbolise its nature and symptoms – as an expression of our subjective experience of life and of our subjectively felt body – 'the lived body'.

No form of conventional medical *testing* however, no matter how technologically sophisticated, can see, scan or diagnose the felt or lived body – nor can it detect a felt sense of *dis-ease* in *that* body – such as a 'broken heart' or a feeling of 'loss of heart'.

Similarly, no form of biomedical *treatment* for hardened arteries can cure 'a hardened heart', just as no form of 'open-heart' surgery can cure someone with 'a closed heart'.

"The heart is often described as a type of pump. With the latest developments in modern technology, there are all kinds of heart operations that can be performed, even the use of heart transplants. In many cases, even when hearts are repaired through medical technology, the same trouble reoccurs at a later date, or the patient recovers only to fall prey to a different, nearly fatal or fatal disease. This is not always the case by any means, but when such a person does recover fully, and maintains good health, it is because [their] beliefs, attitudes and feelings have changed for the better, and because the person 'has a heart' again; in other words because the patient himself has regained the will to live."

"Many people who have heart trouble feel that they have 'lost the heart' for life. They may feel broken-hearted for many reasons. They may feel heartless, or imagine themselves to be so cold-hearted that they punish themselves literally by trying to lose their heart."

"With many people having such difficulties, the addition of love in the environment may work far better than any heart operation. A new pet given to a bereaved individual has saved more people from needing heart operations than any physician. In other words, a 'love transplant' in the environment may work far better overall than a heart-transplant operation, or a bypass, or whatever; in such ways the heart is allowed to heal itself."

"The condition of your heart is affected, for example, by your own feelings about it. If you consider yourself to be cold-hearted or heartless, those feelings will have a significant effect upon that

physical organ. If you feel broken-hearted then you will also have that feeling reflected in one way or another in the physical organ itself.... each individual also has many options open. Everyone who feels broken-hearted does not necessarily die of heart failure for example. The subject of health cannot be considered in an isolated fashion ... each person will try to fulfil their own unique abilities, and to 'fill out' the experience of life as fully as possible."

From Roberts, Jane *The Way Toward Health – A Seth Book*

Case Example 3

A recently bereaved widow, whose husband Harry died from a heart attack, finds herself suffering disturbing chest pains at night and goes to see her physician. The physician sees her symptoms only as signs of some possible organic disorder which might be 'causing' them. He sends her to a consultant to test for possible heart conditions. The tests proving inconclusive, the consultant ends up diagnosing mild angina, and prescribes beta-blockers. These in turn prove to have little effect on the patient's symptoms.

On visiting her physician a second time however, the latter recalls her recent bereavement and, as a result, begins to read the bodily 'text' of her symptoms in a different way, understanding them in the life context of her loss and the pain it may be causing her. Rather than seeking a purely clinical 'diagnosis' of the patient's symptoms he himself listens to his patient in a genuinely patient way. As a result an insight flashes through his mind which he shares with her. He 'sees' that she may be suffering from a doubly *broken heart*: "the one that killed Harry, and the one you're left alive with, that hurts when you're most alone in the middle of the night...the broken heart that gave up and the one that has to carry on painfully." This *heartfelt* hearing of the patient and the *heart-to-heart* talk that ensue are the first time anyone has ever acknowledged the pain of her grief. It gives her the *strength of heart* to acknowledge and bear it in a new way. Her symptoms disappear. The patient's heart symptoms disappear as bodily symbols and metaphorical signifiers of her pained heart, not through an intellectual understanding of their significance alone but through a memory arising from the *feeling heart* of the physician.

This paradigmatic case vignette, cited by Dr David Zigmond in an article on different modes of patient-physician communication, goes to the heart of the contrast between biomedical diagnosis and what could be called 'life diagnosis'.

The root meaning of the term 'diagnosis' actually is 'through knowledge' (*dia-gnosis*). Yet the Greek verb, *gignostikein,* from which the word *gnosis* (knowledge) derives did not mean merely knowledge of or about something – (for example biomedical knowledge of the body). Instead it denoted the sort of knowing we refer to when we speak of being 'familiar' with people, of 'knowing' them well or intimately as human beings – in much the same way that family doctors used to know or be familiar with their patients, as if a part of their families.

It was this type of 'knowing' that the doctor in Zigmond's case study brought to bear in relating to the widow – not just his standard body of medical knowledge 'about' the heart as a biological organ and the type of 'diagnosis' to which it can lead. His method consisted simply of having the patience to listen to his patient in a different way – not seeking a diagnosis of a possible heart 'condition' but affirming her *heartbreak* in a *heartfelt* way. By 'bearing with' his patient in this way, helping to bear the burden of her pained heart with her - she no longer felt herself so painfully alone in bearing it – and was able to find a *new bearing* towards the bereavement that occasioned it.

The paradox that Zigmond notes however, is that despite the inconclusiveness of the initial medical tests, had the physician himself not embodied this new and different bearing towards his patient – had he not heard her in a *heartfelt* way as a human being but simply treated her as a potential 'case' of angina – then the patient herself might well have found herself in the position of having no way to express the heartbreak of her loss *except* through actual and perhaps increasingly acute cardiac symptoms – using her biological heart as an instrument of what Freud called 'organ speech'.

The physician's capacity for a different type of listening – one that did not merely serve as a prelude to some form of purely biomedical diagnosis was therefore 'preventative medicine' in the deepest sense. For it may well have forestalled a process whereby this patient might well have ended up as a genuine 'heart case' requiring serious medical intervention. Alternatively, she might have found herself seen as a so-called 'heart sink' patient - someone who repeatedly 'bothers' her doctor, but whose medical tests continue to reveal no conclusive, measurable signs of any organic disorder or heart disease – thus suggesting some form of malingering. Yet such 'heart-sink' patients are not a marginal group. In their persistence, they are simply unconsciously reacting to the absence of a type of listening that most patients actually seek – the type of listening required for 'life diagnosis' and 'life doctoring'.

This one single case described by Zigmond is therefore 'paradigmatic' – for in its simplicity it nevertheless reveals in full clarity the sharply opposing frameworks or 'paradigms' of Biological Medicine and Life Medicine, Bio-medical Doctoring and Life Doctoring. Indeed recent research has shown that many older widows die within three years of their bereavement – not due to arterial disease but principally through an enlargement of the heart's pumping chamber – in other words a (painfully) 'throbbing heart'.

Zigmond also offers us a study in the very meaning of 'diagnosis' as such – showing how different ways of listening to and coming to 'know' a patient can themselves have a direct bearing on the patient's health and medical condition itself. Our *biology* has its basis in our *biography*, and in that larger *body of awareness* that is our *life world* as a whole. For it is always within the specific contexts of our life world that we experience a felt 'dis-ease', just as it is *capacities of awareness* that allow us to relate to and respond to our life world in a healthy way – *with* awareness.

Illness can and has been understood in many ways: in a purely objective and biomedical way, as a mechanical, neurophysiological 'effect' of psychical stress or trauma, as a relation to our life world and other people in it, as a form of silent bodily *communication* or even protest, as blocked action or communication, and/or as a metaphorical *language* through which we give silent bodily *expression* to any *subjectively* felt 'dis-ease'. Understanding organic illness as a language of awareness embraces all other understandings of it. More importantly it provides us with an understanding of illness that affirms its innate *meaningfulness* in the life of the individual – as an expression and embodiment of their lived experience of themselves and of their life world as a whole, as an expression and embodiment of the degree of awareness they bring to their experience, and as an expression and embodiment too, of the specific capacities or 'organs' of awareness that they do or do not exercise in relating and responding to their experienced self and world – for it is these specific capacities that offer new keys to diagnosing illness *as* a language. (see The Language of Illness and Illness as a Language)

Reference:

Dr David Zigmond, *Three Types of Encounter in the Healing Arts: Dialogue, Dialectic and Didacticism*

Life Medicine and Organic Impairment

It is the organising or 'ordering' capacities of the lived body that allow us not just to remain open to, sense and feel, take and breathe in, digest and metabolise our experience of life but also to:

(a) *make sense* of our lives and life world in an organised and ordered way, and

(b) engage in life and respond to the world in a meaningful and fulfilling way. This is achieved through what the existential physician and neurologist Kurt Goldstein called "ordered performances".

By this he meant ordered activities or patterns of action of any sort that we are normally able to enact within or in response to our life world or environment – whether basic actions such as breathing, moving, walking, talking, clothing ourselves, cooking, eating or fulfilling domestic tasks etc., or more sophisticated 'performances' such as engaging in highly skilled creative, communicative or professional activities and interactions.

Chronic or permanent loss of or impairment to organs and organic functions (for example loss of mobility, sight or hearing) impair and limit such ordered life activities or 'performances'. They also affect and express states of our *organism as a whole* and are felt through 'generalised' organismic states such as fatigue, depression, loss of cognitive capacities or libido etc.

From the perspective of Life Medicine however, to see biological 'death' resulting from organ failure as the end point of our being or existence is to forget that the lived body, being a non-physical body of feeling awareness or soul – our 'soul body' – is by nature eternal.

Therefore what is essentially threatened by a continued or worsening organic impairment – even if 'life threatening' - is not any form of 'absolute death' but rather what is of absolute importance to the current *life* and *health* of the patient in this life and this world i.e. their capacity to *actualise their individual potentials* by means of specific organic capacities and the ordered 'performances' or patterns of action they facilitate. For as Goldstein wrote:

"...health is not an objective condition which can be understood by the methods of natural science alone. It is rather a condition related to the mental attitude by which the individual has to value what is essential for his life. 'Health' appears thus as a value; its value consists in the individual's capacity to actualise his nature to the degree, that for him at least, is essential."

If this understanding offers us a deeper insight into the true essence of 'health', what then are its implications for our understanding of the essence of 'illness'? In the context of organic impairment this question takes us beyond the purely clinical realm of biological medicine and takes us once again into the realm of personal *life meaning.*

For example, a partial loss of movement in a leg may *mean* very little to a sedentary worker but *everything* to an athlete such as a runner or sportsman, just as a speech impairment may mean much less to a manual labourer but everything to a salesman, teacher or writer – inducing an overall organismic reaction that Goldstein calls 'catastrophic' shock and anxiety – being a threat to the very essence of the individual's 'life' or 'existence' understood *as a means of self-actualisation*. On the other hand a patient may be known to have a 'disease' in a potentially 'life threatening' cancer *without this in any way* outwardly affecting their capacity for self-actualisation through specific patterns of action or organised 'performances'. If, as a result of this 'disease' diagnosis however, the life world and life possibilities of the cancer patient are shrunk down to merely being kept alive in a hospital bed and/or subject to hi-tech radiological or chemotherapeutic treatments which radically reduce their quality of life – then it is difficult to argue that this type of 'medicine' in any way benefits their 'health' in the sense defined by Goldstein.

As for illness or 'disease', he writes:

"It may be stated as certain that any disease is an abnormality but not that every abnormality is a disease."

So for example, when people get ill through 'stress' i.e. when demands far beyond what Goldstein calls their "average potentialities" are imposed on them – they may recognise an *abnormality* in their condition, for example feel ill with the symptoms of a cold or flu – *an ailment* – but they do not regard themselves for this reason as having 'a disease'.

In general however, whatever 'symptoms' may be observed, such as high blood pressure, or whatever 'diseases' may be bio-medically diagnosed as a result – for example heart disease – all that has actually occurred is a deviation from a *biological norm*.

Yet this scientific norm may have little to do with a patient's own highly *individual* norm for assessing their own 'health' – understood as their capacity to lead a healthy and fulfilling life.

What biomedicine judges by its own purely *biological norms* to be a 'disease' therefore, is in essence nothing more than an observable *change of state* of the organism, one that may not only be more or less temporary – but also more or less meaningful, threatening or catastrophic to a patient's experience of *life* – not just the life of their physical body.

For as Seth declares:

"The body does not recognise <u>diseases as diseases</u> in usually understood terms. It regards all activity as experience, as a momentary condition of life, as a balancing situation." from *The Way Toward Health* by Jane Roberts

Yet biological medicine understands its primary purpose as to fight disease and prevent death at any cost – qualitative and quantitative - to the life of the patient. This implies that disease is merely and invariably an abnormality with no meaning – and that life itself consists merely in just continuing to 'be alive' or 'survive' biologically, rather than *living* in a way that brings a necessary, minimum degree of self-actualisation and fulfilment (the essence of 'health').

That is why, in cases where a patient is left with a remaining deficit or chronic and incurable organic impairment which more or less severely limits their capacity for a particular type of ordered "performance" or life activity, Goldstein's view was that it was of the utmost importance for the individual to find ways to re-order and if necessary *limit* their life world itself - what he called their "milieu" – not through mere institutionalisation or for the purposes of medical treatment but in a way that:

a) reduces the demands imposed on the individual to respond with "ordered performances" to an extent they are no longer capable of or can cope with

b) nevertheless provides the patient with an ordered environment in which they can still continue to engage in fulfilling forms of ordered activity, old or new.

Though Goldstein dealt with patients suffering from severe neurological damage, this also applies to people with far less severe illnesses or even minor ailments – to which they might respond by taking days off work, staying at home or in bed etc. – all of which are simple ways of temporarily limiting their life world to a less demanding or stressful "milieu" – but one in which they can nevertheless engage in some satisfactory ordered activities or work of some sort.

'Order' is in this way central to Goldstein's view of organic impairment, suggesting a manner in which the physician could serve as a 'life doctor' in the most literal sense – restoring a minimum degree of healthily fulfilling and ordered activity to the patient's *life* and *well-being* rather than seeking only to cure or alleviate a physical disease or impairment.

"...being well means to be capable of ordered behaviour which may prevail in spite of the impossibility of certain performances which were formerly possible. But the new state of health is not the same as the old one ... Recovery is a newly achieved state of ordered functioning ... <u>a new individual norm.</u>"

With this final emphasis, Goldstein affirms that the *new* norm, like the old one, must be an individual one and nothing imposed from without – based on ordered activities satisfying to the individual's essential nature – even if a portion of this 'essence' may have permanently lost its capacity for a full, undefective and ordered expression.

Life Medicine, like the reflections on health and illness that form part of the 'existential neurology' of Goldstein, also affirms the significance of *free choice* on the part of the patient. Thus there may be a situation in which a patient must freely decide whether and to what extent to *either* limit his or her existing life world and its ordered activities in the face of particular limits to their capacities *or* to continue to engage in these activities as before despite the pain or suffering that accompanies them (for example by staying in an over-demanding job).

Whatever the patient decides – with the potential help, encouragement and counselling of the physician as 'life doctor' – the outcome is a way in which the patient freely decides to adapt his or her environment or milieu to his own needs and desires – rather than being forced to adapt *to* them.

Recognising this, we have immediately transcended the one-sided Darwinian notion that organisms survive and thrive solely by *adapting to their environment* - rather than *by adapting that environment* – their life world – in a way that best serves their essential health and well-being.

This is also significant given that most people live in *two* environments or 'life worlds'. One is a 'negative environment' in which social structures and economic conditions actually and constantly deprive individuals of potentials for healthy self-actualisation and instead overload them with demands unrelated to these potentials – often to the point where they cannot 'cope' with these demands or the lack of fulfilment they get from meeting them. As a result people get ill simply by virtue of adapting to a fundamentally unhealthy or sick social-economic environment – and are medically treated simply to restore their capacity to function economically in a way that serves that environment.

The other environment is whatever 'positive' environment, life world or milieu individuals are able to forge for themselves within or outside their 'negative' environment. This positive environment is one that genuinely serves the individual's need to take time, not just for rest, recuperation or distraction from the ills and illnesses induced by their negative environment, but also and above all for activities that serve their positive self-actualisation, and with it their essential *life health* – something that has nothing to do with so-called 'healthy lifestyles'.

Reference: Goldstein, Kurt *The Organism*

Life, Death and 'Terminal Illness'

"The name of the bow is life. Its work is death."

Heraclitus

The Greek word for 'life' (*bios*) also means 'bow'. Yet the apparent truism that life is a span of time drawn out, like the string of a bow, between birth and death, and that the very body that sustains our life will eventually also 'work' our death is one that most people would like to forget. Their belief in biological medicine is not just rooted in a quasi-religious respect for the authority of modern science and technology and its medical application. In many cases, it is also rooted in the false belief that birth and death are the alpha and omega of our existence as such i.e. that death brings a final end to our lives, to our consciousness – indeed to our very being – rather than releasing us, like a bow releases an arrow, into different and broader dimensions of existence, consciousness and life. This belief in turn is linked to the modern scientific notion that consciousness is a mere product or property of our bodies and brains – a notion that is actually quite illogical. For given that we only *know* we exist or have a body through a (conscious) *awareness* of being and of having a body, to reduce this *awareness* of our bodies to some product or property *of* our bodies, is like reducing our entire *dream awareness* to the product or property of some particular thing we are aware of dreaming.

As for what we think of as our bodies themselves, there is not an atom in them that does not itself 'survive' the disintegration of the human organism – or is not imbued with its own consciousness. Yet the body that concerns us here is not what we think of as our 'mortal' or 'physical' body but rather what in Life Medicine goes by the name of the 'lived' or 'felt body'. Since this body is essentially nothing but a *body of consciousness,* a distinct 'psychic body' or 'soul body', it cannot but survive the disintegration of our physical body and its soul – made up of atomic and molecular consciousness.

For centuries however, the understanding that the soul itself has its own innate bodily shape and form – its *own* body - has been surrendered to a false separation of 'body' and 'mind' – or 'body' and 'soul'. Paradoxically therefore, whereas most people believe that the possibility of life after death depends on the body and soul being separate entities, in a sense the very opposite is the case – the soul survives death by virtue of having its own body. Proof of the 'existence' of such a body requires no supposedly 'scientific' form of experimentation or evidence, nor even the experience of dreaming or so-called 'out of body' states in which we inhabit another, entirely subjective body. For in reality this felt body or 'soul body' – the body as we subjectively feel and experience it – is and can be the *only body* that we ever experience. Its existence is therefore 'empirically' self-evident and not an hypothesis to be proven.

Even putting such philosophical arguments aside however, the fact remains that the very *belief* that death marks the ultimate terminus or end point of our being and consciousness is in many cases a principal reason why so many people with actual or potentially 'terminal' illnesses resort to biomedical treatments. For if death truly is the terminal point of our existence, then it will seem to them that their 'life' depends on such treatments, i.e. life and being *as such* and not just their existence in *this life*. So for them any medical means of forestalling death or extending their current life is understandably attractive to them – even if it comes at the expense of further *weakening* their own bodies through treatments such as invasive surgery, radiotherapy or chemotherapy, and/or severely reducing their quality of life through other side effects of such treatments.

That is why another important role of the Life Doctor is to help patients come to more deeply considered decisions about whether or not to accept the forms of biomedical treatment that may be recommended to them – often with considerable pressure. Above all, however, the Life Doctor must be able to reassure the patient with *absolute personal and philosophical conviction* that *no one* - whether seemingly healthy or severely ill – dies before they are inwardly ready to die for some reason connected with their current life and existence in all its dimensions – and not just the life of 'the body' as biological medicine understands it.

"... no person dies ahead of his or her time. The individual chooses the time of death. It is true however, that many cancers and conditions such as AIDS result because the immunity system has been so tampered with that the body has not been allowed to follow through with its own balancing act." Seth, in *The Way Toward Health* by Jane Roberts (see Appendix)

"Again, however, no individual dies of cancer or AIDS, or any other condition, until they themselves have set the time."

Seth also adds the following insights, all of which form part of the philosophical framework of Life Medicine and Life Doctoring:

"People with life-threatening diseases ... often feel that further growth, development, or expansion are highly difficult, if not impossible to achieve at a certain point in their lives. Often there are complicated family relationships that the person does not know how to handle ... In all cases, however, the need for value fulfilment, expression, and creativity are so important to life that when these are threatened, life itself is at least momentarily weakened. Innately, each person does realise that there is life after death, and in some instances such people realise that it is indeed time to move to another level of reality, to die and set out again with another brand new world ... Often, seriously ill people quite clearly recognise such feelings but they have been taught not to speak of them. The desire to die is considered cowardly, even evil, by some religions – and yet behind that desire lies all of the vitality of the will to life, which may already be seeking new avenues of expression and meaning."

An important role of the Life Doctor in relation to so-called 'terminal illness' should therefore be to question how the very term 'terminal' is understood by the patient – in other words whether they themselves see death as an absolute termination of their being or can understand it as a return and transition of the soul to a "brand new world", i.e. a different dimension of consciousness in which possibilities of expression, growth and development frustrated in their current life and world might be fulfilled. For behind the 'will to die' do not necessarily lie 'suicidal' impulses in the way they are ordinarily understood – as the expression of a desire to annihilate the self. Such impulses may also arise from a conscious or unconscious recognition of what the world to come offers the self in terms of greater fulfilment. This recognition is important in another way too – since many suicides would be avoided were the individual to realise that death does *not* bring an end to their life – or to important challenges not met within it.

As Seth points out, it is a scientific dogma *"...that life is meaningless, that it has no purpose, and that its multitudinous parts fell together through the workings of chance alone..."* adding that *"such dogma is far more religious than scientific, for it also expects to be believed without proof, on faith alone. All of life is seen as heading for extinction in any case. The entire concept of a soul, life after death, or even life from one generation to the next, becomes doubtful, to say the least ... In such a philosophical world it would seem that man has no power at all... those concepts can have a hand in the development of would-be suicides, particularly of a young age, for they seem to effectively block a future."*

This question of 'life after death' then is by no means 'merely' metaphysical or philosophical, for every individual bears within them a set of philosophical beliefs or assumptions with a profound bearing on their relation not just to health and illness, but to the relation of medicine to life and death.

"There are those who come down with one serious disease – say heart trouble – who are cured through a heart transplant or other medical procedure, only to fall prey to another, seemingly unrelated disease, such as cancer. It would relieve the

minds of family and friends, however if they understood that the individual involved did not 'fall prey' to the disease, and that he or she was not a victim in <u>usual</u> terms ... This does not mean that anyone consciously decides to get such-and-such a disease, but it does mean that some people instinctively realise that their own development <u>does</u> now demand another new framework of existence."

"Much loneliness results when people who know they are going to die feel unable to communicate with loved ones for fear of hurting their feelings. Still other kinds of individuals will live long productive lives even while their physical mobility or health is most severely impaired. They will still feel that they had work to do, or that they were needed ..."

Specifically with regard to cancer, Seth comments that:

"Many cancer patients have martyr-like characteristics, often putting up with undesirable situations or conditions for years. They feel powerless, unable to change, yet unwilling to stay in the same position. The most important point is to arouse such a person's belief in his or her strength and power. In many instances these people shrug their shoulders, saying "What will happen, will happen," but they do not physically struggle against their [life] situation."

"It is ... vital that these patients are not overly medicated, for oftentimes the side effects of some cancer-eradicating drugs are dangerous in themselves. There has been some success with people who imagine that the cancer is instead some hated enemy or monster or foe, which is then banished with mental mock battles over a period of time. While the technique does have its

advantages, it also pits one portion of the self against the other." [my stress]

"Cancer patients most usually feel an inner impatience as they sense their own need for future expansion and development, only to feel it thwarted." [my stress]

"Again, we cannot generalise overmuch, but many persons <u>know quite well that they are not sure whether they want to live or die.</u> The overabundance of cancer cells represents nevertheless the need for expression and expansion – the only arena left open – or so it would seem."

The phrases I have italicised above offer important insights that Life Doctoring for patients with potentially terminal illnesses needs to take account of.

On the one hand, they affirm the general understanding of Life Medicine that in seeking to 'fight', 'conquer' or 'get rid of' an illness, one is effectively trying to fight, conquer or get rid of a vital part of ourselves – a part that is showing us how 'sick' or ill-at-ease we are with our lives or way of living – and that in a very specific way for which the timing and specific nature of our illness will always offer us clear clues.

On the other hand, they return us again to fundamental issues of life and death – or rather beliefs regarding them. For, if death is seen as the final end of life and being, then there might not only be an understandable *impatience* both to 'cure' any disease we believe can or will kill us – regardless of our will to live - but perhaps also an impatience to 'live life to the full' in whatever limited period of time we believe (or are led to believe) we still have. This again is understandable, and yet there is also the possibility that this intense impatience to 'make the best use' of our remaining years or 'live them to the full' (whether we are healthy or ill) may be a concealed expression of a still unacknowledged *will to die* – expressed through an impatient desire to get through these years not just as intensely but also as *quickly* as possible.

Another important key to Life Doctoring for 'life-threatening' illness is therefore *patience as such*. That is because for whatever reasons and in whatever ways an individual may have become or continues to remain 'a patient' – this may be a result either of them being *too patient* with their life circumstances or too *impatient* to deal with them except through illness, biomedical treatments – or even an exaggerated 'will to live'. For through this will to live some 'patients' *may* be seeking to impatiently hide from a still unacknowledged 'will to die' – or to impatiently *deny* any remaining inner conflict between their will to live and their will to die. This dilemma becomes even more charged as a 'life or death issue' if a patient is or feels pressured to quickly decide for example, whether to *immediately accept* potentially dangerous forms of biomedical testing and treatment – or simply *to be patient* – not just to 'wait and see' but to give themselves time to see more deeply into themselves, their life and their illness. At such times it might well be of great importance for 'the patient' to heed the words of Martin Heidegger: *"Patience is the truly human mode of being."*

Reference: Roberts, Jane *The Way Toward Health - a Seth book*

Life Medicine and the Secret of Longevity

'Longevity' is usually understood as living for a long time. Yet one can live for a 100 years or more and still lead a life dominated by 'time poverty' and/or lacking in 'quality time'. And being too busy to experience life in all its richness, depth and fullness – and to draw meaning and fulfilment from it – is itself a major cause of illness. In contrast to the association of 'life' itself with permanent activity and 'busy-ness', Life Medicine recognises that the true 'length' of our lives has less to do with the mere quantity of years we live than with the quality and extent of the time we *take for ourselves* and others whilst living them. Indeed *taking time* – by which I mean 'taking our own time' – is the true secret of health and longevity in *every sense* – both qualitative and quantitative. A life lived more slowly – given more time – is both a richer and a longer life. The key to this in turn is *making time* or *taking time* for ourselves, for others – and for all the things listed below – and many more:

Taking time to feel and be more aware of our bodies *all the time* – and not just when we are ill.

Taking time to feel and be more aware of our bodies *as a whole* – and not the just the parts of them we are using or feeling *at any given time*.

Taking time to be aware of our *breathing* – and to consciously breathe more slowly.

Taking time to be more aware of our *speaking* – and to consciously speak more slowly.

Taking time to feel our thoughts and feelings more deeply *before* we speak them.

Taking time to feel and adjust our posture and to relax our muscles *before* speaking or moving.

Taking time to allow longer intervals of silence in communication – intervals in which we take all the time we need to silently take in and digest what another person has said *before* reacting to it.

Taking time to premeditate any activities *before* we engage in them, to choose and *time* our actions and interactions in a way that feels right in our bodies – neither needlessly rushing or delaying them – and *never* just 'going from one thing to another' in time.

Taking time to *pause* and *stop time* – to create 'breathing spaces' between *every single* interaction, task or activity we engage in – time to rest from them, to recollect, digest and process our experience of them, to feel for deeper layers of meaning in them - and let fresh insights arise from them.

Taking time to feel for and return to a place of deep inner stillness and silence within us before our next actions or words – so that we act and speak from that place of inner stillness and silence.

Taking time to 'open ourselves' bodily – to feel and take in the entire space around our bodies.

Taking time to 'ground ourselves' bodily – to feel the ground beneath our feet and our entire lower body below the waist.

Taking time to 'centre' both ourselves and our breathing in our true spiritual and physical centre of gravity - our lower abdomen – using *only* our abdominal muscles to breathe and feeling the inner space of the abdomen as the true seat and centre of both our body and self.

Taking time to 'body' what we feel before expressing or acting on our feelings – for example to find a tone of voice, facial expression or look in our eyes that truly fits the way we feel inside.

Taking time to make wordless feeling contact with others before speaking with them – to feel and take another person in as 'some body' and not just an 'other mind' or 'talking head'.

Taking time to 'come to our senses' – using our bodies to experience more vividly and intensely the immediate sensory and sensuous dimension of every encounter or experience, person or place, thought or emotion, situation or state of being.

Taking time to be with and 'bear with' ourselves and others in 'pregnant silence' – thus allowing new ways of feeling ourselves and relating to others – a new 'inner bearing' – to be born from that pregnant silence.

Taking time in all these ways – not just to *slow down* but also to *savour* time – to let every single experienced life activity, event or encounter *linger on* in our bodies and *fill them* with felt and *living meaning*.

Taking time in this way to experience true inner 'full-fillment' in life - rather than trying to just 'lead a full life'.

Taking time to be truly *patient* with our bodies, our feelings and our lives – and in this way both deepen and stretch out *time itself* – rather than becoming 'a patient' or seeking to 'extend' our life.

'The Secret of Longevity' – taking more time in one's life to be more aware of *time itself* – and to *linger* in a bodily way with all that occurs within it.

PART 4

DISTINCTIONS CENTRAL TO LIFE MEDICINE

Basic Distinctions

Life Medicine is rooted in a number of new and fundamental distinctions.

1. Between feeling ill and 'getting ill'.
2. Between feeling ill-at-ease with one's life and being 'ill'.
3. Between the particular life meaning of an illness for the individual and its biological 'causes'.
4. Between our subjectively 'felt body' or 'lived body' and the 'clinical body' or 'physical' body.
5. Between the body as an embodiment of the human *being* and the body as a biological *machine*.
6. Between our subjectively felt sense of bodily 'dis-ease' and an 'objective' bio-medically diagnosed 'disease'.
7. Between seeing the patient's life problem *as their illness* and seeing the patient's illness as the symptom of a *life problem*.
8. Between talking to a doctor *because* one is ill and getting ill in order to talk to a doctor.
9. Between seeing illness itself *as a symptom* and seeing symptoms only as possible *signs of an illness*.
10. Between knowing that one may die *by means* of an illness and believing that one dies simply 'from' an illness.
11. Between *meditating* an illness to heal one's life and *medicating* an illness to heal one's body.
12. Between seeing a patent's illness as something to be cured and understanding that *the illness is there to cure the patient* – to help them to heal and transform their lives.

Table of Differences:
Biological Medicine versus Life Medicine

Assumptions of Biological Medicine	Basic Principles of Life Medicine
The purpose of medicine is to *cure the illness.*	The purpose of illness is to *cure the patient.*
The illness is the enemy.	The illness is the cure.
Health is 'good'. Illness is 'bad'.	Illness is part of a healthy life, just as dealing with life-problems is.
Health and illness are opposites.	Illness is a natural part of a healthy life.
The *human body* can be separated from the life of the individual *human being.*	The human body is a *living embodiment* of the individual human being.
The patient's life problem is their *illness* and its symptoms.	The patient's illness is the symptom of a *life problem.*
Illnesses are *things* that we 'get' or 'have'.	Illnesses are natural life and learning *processes.*
Illnesses have 'causes' but no *life meaning* - aside from interfering with our lives and thus requiring treatment.	Illnesses have *life meanings* – symbolising, and thus helping us explore important life questions.
A somatic symptom is a diagnostic 'sign' of a bodily disease.	A symptom is a somatic *symbol* of a felt *dis-ease.*
Diagnosis identifies *independent disease entities* in the body and thus guides treatment.	There are *no such things* as disease entities separable from the body and life of the individual as whole.

Illness can be life-threatening and thus a cause of death. People die *from* illness if they are untreated or incurable.	People die *through* illnesses and not 'from' or 'of' them – and do so only if they are *ready to die.*
The aim of medicine is to 'cure' or rid ourselves of an illness.	The illness itself is the potential 'cure' – helping to heal or 'make whole' our self.
Illness is an *attack* by 'foreign bodies' or 'non-self' organisms such as viruses or mutated cells.	Illness is a form of *pregnancy* – the bodily expression of unborn aspects of our self as a whole.
Medicine is *war* against disease - helping our bodies to 'fight' disease.	Medicine is *midwifery* – helping us to give birth to a new sense of self.
Healing means bringing about changes *in our bodies.*	Healing means *letting our bodies change us* - our bodily sense of self.
Mind and body 'affect' one another though physiological processes.	Every bodily or somatic state *is* a state of consciousness – and vice versa.
Illness is the result of an *objective* biological process occurring in the *physical body.*	Illness is the result of changes occurring in our subjective or *felt body* – which is also our bodily identity, our 'body self'.
Feeling ill results from 'getting ill' with some objective physical 'disease'.	'Getting ill' results from feeling ill – from a subjectively felt *dis-ease.*
The way we feel our bodies – our inwardly felt body – is a subjective expression of the physical body.	The physical body is an outward expression of our subjective body – our inwardly felt body.

The aim of the physician is to help the patient to recover or 'feel themselves' again – to feel the same way they did before getting ill.	The aim of the physician is to help the patient to change – to feel a different self to the one they felt before getting ill.
The purpose of the physician-patient relationship is to heal the patient by diagnosing and treating their symptoms.	It is the *relationship itself* that is the chief healing factor, helping – or not helping - the patient to heal.
The health of the individual is an entirely private matter and a function of their bodies.	Individual health is an expression of the health of *human relations* in society. Sicknesses are sicknesses of relation.
Symptoms are caused by a *physical disease* or disorder in the *human body or brain.*	Both symptoms and their causes are the expression of a *felt dis-ease* of the individual *human being.*
Symptoms have bodily *causes.*	Symptoms are bodily *symbols.*
The human body is a *functioning biological machine.*	The human body is a *living biological language.*
We 'have' a body – a body which we can feel in different ways.	We do not 'have' a body. We *body* – *embodying* the way we feel.
Health is our capacity to maintain a *fully functioning* body and mind, no matter how sick the society in which we live.	Health is our capacity to *fully embody* and *fulfil* our values and potentials as individual human beings.
Every patient's illness is just an individual 'case' of a generic disease.	Every patient's illness is a unique expression of their individuality.

Medical science is based on 'proven facts', such as the way the immune system functions.	Modern medicine is based on *linguistic metaphors* – such as the *military* metaphor of immune 'defences'.
Most medical research is 'neutral' and 'objective'.	Most medical research is profit driven and biased by corporate funding.
Most medications are scientifically trialled and tested to show their effectiveness and safety.	Most medications are little more effective than placebos, whilst often producing severe or even life-threatening side effects.
Modern biomedical treatments of illness save countless lives and are therefore indispensable.	Statistics from recognised medical journals in the U.S.A. show that biomedical treatments are themselves *the third principal cause of death* after cancer and heart disease – if not *the* leading cause of death as well as countless *iatrogenic* (medically induced) illnesses and symptoms.
Inner well-being is an expression of the health of the body.	The health of the body is an expression of inner well-being.

Life Medicine and 'Alternative Medicine'

One of the principal attractions of 'alternative' forms of medicine is that its practitioners tend to give a lot more time to their patients than doctors – at least in the initial consultation – and to ask questions about their lives and life situation as a whole of a sort that biomedical doctors have no time or see no point in. All the more disappointing then, that such initial consultations usually prove to be a mere *prelude* to a procedure identical in principle to that of any biomedical doctor i.e. internally framing and 'diagnosing' the patient's bodily symptoms in terms of an unquestioned body of knowledge (for example homeopathy or Traditional Chinese Medicine) and then prescribing some form of pre-given remedy or engaging in some form of pre-prescribed alternative 'treatment' – all in a way that the practitioner has been *taught* is appropriate to the patient's condition according to their training – and which therefore demands of them no further or deeper thought.

The effectiveness of the alternative remedies or treatments is in large part due to the *relationship* of trust established between practitioner and patient and to their joint *belief* in the rationale and efficacy of whatever remedy or operational procedure (for example a selected acupunctural procedure) is prescribed. Belief and trust are the real foundation of the so-called 'placebo effect' – though this is a no less important factor in the efficacy of much orthodox biomedical practice than it is in the practice of alternative medicine. For even so-called random double-blind drug trials designed to exclude subjective or observational bias on the part of *both* patient and researcher assume in advance that the patient's own body is *not itself aware* of whether it has been given a 'placebo' or a complex pharmaceutical drug even though the latter, is bound to be registered and reacted to by the body and registered by the patient in one way or another.

The term 'alternative medicine' belongs to a variety of so-called approaches to medicine regarded as 'holistic' – that claim to 'treat' the person and not just the disease, i.e. the human being as a 'whole' and not just their body. Yet the very language of medicine and of holistic healing – in particular the use of the little word 'and' in stock phrases such as 'mind *and* body', 'body *and* soul' or 'body, mind *and* spirit' effectively reduces the human being to a mere assemblage of separate parts. In this way holistic medicine is again, no different in essence from biological medicine – with which it also shares the *same basic aim* of seeking 'causes' and 'cures' for illness rather than exploring its life meaning for the patient. Indeed the term 'holistic healing' does not even make linguistic sense, for it constitutes what is called a pleonasm like 'black darkness'. That is because the words 'whole' and 'holistic' actually share many of the same roots as the word 'healing' itself – for example the Middle English *hole/hoole* and *hāl* from which the words 'hail' – meaning 'be blessed with long life' – 'hale' and 'healthy' are derived. In its linguistic roots, therefore, the phrase 'holistic healing' means nothing more than 'healing which makes healthy'.

On the other hand, alternative methods of healing such as acupressure, acupuncture and different types of massage can certainly be understood as stimulating a type of healing *inter-cellular communication* between different organs and parts of the body – not through the flow of any 'thing' that might be called 'energy' but rather in the form of breath or air-like flows of atomic, molecular and cellular awareness. Understanding such flows in this way can help bring us to closer to the real but as-yet unexplored essence of what is called 'alternative medicine' and its distinction from both Biological Medicine and Life Medicine – namely that it works *neither* through the so-called 'physical body' nor through any form of 'energy body' but rather through a bounded portion of our larger 'body of awareness' or 'psychic body' that could be called the 'physical soul'.

Our felt or lived body could, in contrast, be called our 'psychic body'. That is because it is essentially the body of our feeling awareness – of our soul or *psyche*. Its field of awareness however, is nothing bounded or contained within the flesh but embraces the entire world around us – our entire *life world* and all we experience within it. What could be called the 'physical soul' on the other hand, is only that limited and 'physically' bounded *portion* of our larger 'psychic body' or 'body of awareness' which takes the form of the human organism – being made up specifically of organised fields units, patterns and flows of *atomic, molecular, cellular* and *organic awareness.* Of these, most people are only indirectly or subconsciously aware. Given this fact however, 'alternative medicine' can be said to replace a *fully conscious and intentional* exploration of the links between illness and life (of the sort that lies at the foundation of 'Life Medicine' and Life

Doctoring) with a focus on removing bodily symptoms of a life 'dis-ease' in a *subconscious or unconscious* way – specifically by seeking to prevent or stop this lived dis-ease working *from* the 'psychic body' and *through* the 'physical soul' into expression as symptoms and illnesses of the 'physical body'. Understood in this way, alternative medicine in all its forms may indeed be effective in ameliorating or working on *symptoms* in a way that does not rely on dangerous forms of biomedical testing and treatment. Yet even though biomedicine recognises neither a psychical 'body of awareness' nor a 'physical soul' made up of organised patterns of atomic, molecular and cellular awareness, the 'effectiveness' of alternative medicine tends to be assessed – even by its own practitioners – *in exactly the same terms as biomedicine.* That is why this 'effectiveness' can and often is disputed or dismissed on the basis of the purely statistical or so-called 'evidence-based' criteria of biomedical science and research, which (like the alternative medicine) fails to research and assess what is most important of all, i.e. the specific *life meaning* of a given symptom or illness for an individual patient as opposed to its supposedly universal 'causes' or 'cures' and the impersonal, statistical evidence surrounding or supporting them.

Biomedicine and alternative medicine differ essentially only in the *language* they use to describe such 'causes' and in the 'cures' they offer. Thus whereas a biomedical practitioner may seek the causes of a disease in our genes or in organic disorders, a practitioner of alternative medicine may seek them in the form of 'blockages' in 'energy flows', an imbalance of so-called 'energy centres' or 'chakras', a lack of specific vitamins or nutrients, or a surfeit of 'bad' ones. And whereas a biomedical practitioner may prescribe a pharmaceutical drug with serious side effects or invasive and potentially dangerous operative surgery as a 'cure', the alternative practitioner merely offers a different form of 'cure' in the form, say, of a natural herb or a safer type of operational procedure such as acupuncture.

Etymological note 1 - on the terms 'whole' and 'heal'

It is a common but false belief that the root meaning of the verb 'to heal' is to 'make whole'. It is true that the word *holistic* comes from the Greek *holos* meaning entire or 'whole'. The word *whole* itself however, comes from Middle English *hole/hoole or hāl* – meaning not only 'healthy' but also 'sound' – as in the German words *Hall* ('echoing sound') and *gesund* – 'healthy' – but also in the sense of a gathering (*ge-*) of 'sound' (*-sund*) as in *a hall* - German *Halle*. A hall is a place of shelter but one that also echoes, reverberates and resounds (German *hallen*). All these English and Germanic words connected with what is 'whole', 'hale' or 'healthy' are thus also intimately related to the German words *heilig/das Heilige* and their English equivalents – *holy* and *the holy* – which in turn refer not just to what is divine or sacred, but also and at the same time that which silently *sounds and resounds* through all that is. Hence the English *hale* and German *heil*, to be in 'sound' health. Hence also the German greeting *Heil!* and English *hail!* – greeting sounds that offer a divine blessing, grant good fortune, salvation and wish the other a long life – and that are echoed today in the everyday greeting words *hello* (English) and *hallo* (German). The German verb *heilen* and English *to heal* – originally meaning to 'protect', 'redeem' or 'save', are all rooted in the Germanic *hailaz* – meaning a sounded magical or sacred blessing, and go back to the Indo-European *kail*. The opposite of all that is sound and hale is what in German is called *das Unheil* – usually translated as 'misfortune', 'calamity', 'catastrophe' or 'disaster'. Yet what sort of 'calamity' or 'catastrophe' is meant here? One that merely causes or results from some sort of accidental misfortune – as illness or ill-health is thought to do. Surely not, since the word *Unheil* has related senses of something being not only unhealthy or unholy but also *unsound*. 'To heal' then, is not simply to restore health in the sense of curing or eliminating a disease but rather to restore the essence of health as 'soundness' or *Ge-sundheit* – to restore *resonance*. For where there is no longer any felt sense of resonance with another human being, how can the human being once again be brought into resonance with the holy - that which shelters and speaks to all beings within the cosmos, understood as a 'hall' or 'house' of God? That is why holy caves and temples were the first places people went to for 'healing'. It is also why the vocations of 'holy man', 'shaman' or 'priest' on the one hand - guardian of a holy cave, hall or temple – and healer on the other, were originally one. The holy man (or woman) was also a human being who effectively worked their capacity (*energein*) to use *holy* sounds and speech in the form of syllables, spells, mantras or prayers to heal – these being sounds and speech *in resonance* with the divine soul of the human being.

Life Medicine and 'Energy Medicine'

"Science is the new religion."

Martin Heidegger

What might be called 'energeticism' has long become the new 'materialism' – an insight that nicely equates with Einstein's famous mathematical equation of energy and matter. In the specific context of Oriental or Indian philosophies and healing practices the only way to do full justice to these traditions would therefore be by first of all freeing them from the imposition of Western and specifically Greek or Latin-derived concepts.

That is why, in almost all 'alternative' or 'New Age' forms of healing that are offered in place of biological medicine, one word is religiously worshipped above all. This is the scientific-sounding word 'energy' – as used in the terms 'energy medicine' and 'energy body'. Through the use of the term energy deference is made to a central term in the religion of modern science – yet without any attempt to define or question what exactly is meant by this term – what 'energy' essentially *is*. Behind this lack of basic questioning lies ignorance of both the linguistic and historic roots of the word 'energy' – for example the fact that this term 'energy' was first promoted in the 19th century by a group of well-known scientists called 'energeticists' who wanted to place the term at the top of the ladder of scientific terms – even though its modern scientific use bears no relation whatsoever either to its roots in the Greek language *or* to the vocabulary of *any* ancient 'spiritual' or 'healing' tradition, Eastern or Western.

The terms 'energy' and 'energy medicine' are as questionable as the term 'holistic medicine' – not least as applied to Oriental forms of medicine such as acupuncture, Chi Gong or Reiki – all of which translate the Chinese term *Chi/Qi* and the Japanese term *Ki* using a modern-scientific term derived from Greek – 'energy'. As for speaking of *Chi/Qi* or *Ki* as some sort of 'energy flow' through the body (for example through so-called 'meridian' lines) this also makes no linguistic sense, since ideograms for *Chi/Qi* and *Ki*, like the Greek word for 'soul' – *psyche* – do *not* refer to any form or flow of 'energy' but to breath – 'the breath of life'. It can be argued then, that what, in terms of Oriental healing traditions, is *today* named 'energy' (or regarded as some form of 'life force') is essentially a breath or air-like flow of *awareness* – for example to a particular point or points in the body where pressure is applied or acupuncture needles are inserted. Yet the problem with *all* forms of so-called 'energy medicine' is that if we look at the original meaning of those Greek words from which the term 'energy' is derived, it make no sense to speak, for example of 'working' in any way 'on' or with someone's 'energy'. For one of the most basic root meanings of the word 'energy' *is* purely and simply *to be engaged in work*.

Today however, to even question the use of the now taken-for-granted and sacrosanct term 'energy' is seen as heretical in the pseudo-science of 'energy medicine', just as it is in the orthodox science of biomedicine. So it needs to be repeated again and again that simply to speak of 'working' with 'energy' in any context – scientific, psychotherapeutic, medical or quasi-medical – is a *distortion* of the root Greek verb *energein* – which means nothing more than simply *'to be engaged in a work'* or *'to actualise something'*. And that given its specifically *Greek* roots the term 'energy' is *least of all* applicable in translating terms such as *Chi*/QI or *Ki* that are central to Chinese and Japanese forms of healing such as *Chi Gong* or *Reiki*.

The danger however, is that many of the ritualised or highly *systematised* bodies of knowledge that sprang from different healing 'traditions' of the past block all fresh exploration, not only of their own root terms, but also of the *root experiences* from which these traditions first arose and took shape. The result is that even highly trained and qualified practitioners or 'masters' of such traditions rarely seek to explore more deeply how and in what manner their own practices and procedures are inwardly *felt* rather than 'proven' to be 'effective' – not just by patients but by the practitioners themselves. Indeed most practitioners of traditional Chinese or Ayurvedic medicine do not even think of asking themselves from what sort of direct, inwardly felt and lived experience of the body such traditions actually arose in the first place – and *before* they were systematised into unquestioned 'bodies of knowledge', or systematised into ritualised practices and procedures. They do not ask, for example, how and in what manner the Chinese sages first came to subjectively sense – through their own 'psychic body' and 'physical soul' – what later came to be called 'meridians' or 'acupuncture points'? Instead, both what I term the 'psychic body' and the 'physical soul' have itself been theoretically *objectified* as some sort of vaguely or wholly undefined 'subtle body' or 'energy body'.

The use in alternative medicine of terms such as 'energy', 'energy body' and 'energy medicine' therefore, continues to play a central role in substituting for and preventing a new type of living, experiential or 'phenomenological' research into the *essence* of many traditional forms of healing, i.e. research aimed at experientially rediscovering and reconceiving the essential *phenomena* involved. Instead, such terms as 'energy' or 'life force' offer authoritative scientific-sounding 'placeholders' for the possible results of such research. The result however, is that no progress is made towards a *radical rethinking* of different traditional healing systems and practices; 'radical' because it truly returns to the *roots* of those traditions – bodily, experiential, historical and linguistic. So it is that what today is misleadingly called 'Energy Medicine' has become the pseudo-scientific New Age substitute for 'Existential Medicine' or 'Life Medicine'.

Yet only the latter can be said to be truly 'holistic' and also in resonance with the different root meanings of the term 'energy'. That is because Life Medicine is based on the recognition that 'to heal' means to address the actually experienced *life* of the human being as a whole – and the way it does or does not *actualise* and fulfil the latent *capacities* or *potentials* of the individual – work or action which effectively actualises specific potentials or capacities being another important root meaning of the term 'energy' itself.

'Life Medicine' therefore, most certainly does *not* constitute yet another of the countless forms of 'alternative' medicine – traditional or 'New Age' – currently promoted on the ever-expanding marketplace of medical practices. Similarly, a 'Life Doctor' is not simply some sort of practitioner of alternative medicine who has been indoctrinated through training in an alternative body of medical 'knowledge' – or who merely uses more 'natural' drugs or safer operative procedures to work 'on' a patient's body. Instead, it is the Life Doctor's own carefully cultivated capacity to directly sense and *resonate* with the *lived body* and *life* of the patient as a whole – and in this way come to understand the inner connections between their illness and their life – that counts most of all in the practice of Life Doctoring and shapes its methods.

As for those who claim that evidence for an 'energy body' exists by virtue of the ability of some people to perceive a colourful 'aura' around the 'physical body', this only goes to show their ignorance of the true nature of the inwardly felt or lived body as a 'body of feeling awareness'. For those who *see* what they think of as a multi-coloured 'energetic' aura show only their inability to directly sense and *feel* the tonal colourations of awareness or 'mood colours' that make up our lived body – and that emanate from and are sensed by every human being not just by trained 'clairvoyants' or 'experts' in 'energy medicine'. What use is it to merely 'see' a colour field around a person's body if one cannot directly and empathically feel and *sense* the tone, quality and 'colour' of their mood as it shows itself directly in their comportment and emanates directly as a mood. For a practitioner of 'energy medicine' to then have to rely on colour charts that 'explain' how *seeing* a particular colour such as red in someone's 'aura' might, for example, 'mean' that this person has 'anger' in them, only goes to show how little capacity that practitioner has to attune to and *sense* another person's mood or feelings directly.

Etymological note 2 - on the roots of the term 'energy'

What unites all the following Greek roots of the word 'energy' are meanings to do with the 'actualisation' or 'working' of potentials or 'powers' (Greek *dynamis*). Thus the Greek *ergon* was used to refer to any type of work. *Energein* meant action or work which is effective and productive of a result. *Energeia* refers to a state of 'being-in-action' or 'being engaged in work'. So to speak of working 'on' or 'with' a person's 'energy' is a pleonasm. It amounts to saying you are working on the action or work they are engaged in. Aristotle also uses the term *energeia* to refer to specific states of consciousness or qualities of awareness associated with 'being in action' or 'being engaged in effective work' – happiness for example. The words *energes/energos* meant 'powerful' and were used to describe powerful siege weapons for example. *Energema* refers to activity which is an expression or embodiment of a potential, 'capacity' or 'capability'. It also means simply a working 'operation' or 'procedure' such as those carried out in surgery - or acupuncture – so again it makes no sense of that procedure working with or 'on' 'energy'. *Energeitai* refers in the New Testament to the working of divine or supernatural powers (*energemat*a) through human action (New Testament). *Energoumene* refers to action (such as prayer) set in operation and empowered by the divine (New Testament). *Energesen* – things *worked* or 'wrought' by God (Old Testament).

Life Medicine and 'Spiritual Healing'
– The Man Who Didn't Want to See

No form of medicine can guarantee a 'cure' for any illness – not least one whose basic principle is that 'the illness is the cure'. The types of truly effective self-healing that Life Doctoring can aid in therefore also require a readiness on the part of the individual patient to alter deep-seated and fundamental *beliefs* about the nature of medicine, health, illness and healing – and to concentrate *primarily* on attaining insights into the meaning of their illness rather than seeking to get rid of it through either conventional or alternative forms of medical treatment. This readiness to alter basic beliefs and interest in understanding both themselves and their illness more deeply may not always be present in the patient. If they also lack experience of any form of inter-personal counselling or therapy – or even have a negative view of it – such a readiness and interest may also be difficult to cultivate. Nevertheless, the importance of the type of insight into the meaning of an individual's illness that Life Medicine offers can even be exemplified by precisely this kind of unready patient, unwilling to see or change their fixed beliefs.

Case Example 4

The patient had, since 2003, been suffering from progressively worsening vision due to a retinal detachment in both eyes. Still being able to read, though only with a magnifier and book rest and more slowly and not as easily as someone with healthy eyes, Life Doctoring was conducted on a correspondence basis.

The Life Doctor was first contacted by the patient by e-mail for three reasons. Firstly, because the patient had exhausted all options offered by conventional medicine, secondly, because out of despair the patient had sought out a spiritual healer and tried alternative methods of healing (one of which promised cellular regeneration of the retina) and, thirdly, because the patient saw in the Life Doctor someone who, as a practitioner of a new form of yoga, could help him as a spiritual teacher and healer on his spiritual 'quest'. This was a quest not just for 'enlightenment' but also to develop superhuman yogic powers or *siddhis* – including not only powers of levitation but also and above all the power to heal his eyes himself.

Below I cite two of his own descriptions of his sight disorder and its relation to both the 'spiritual quest' it triggered and his notion of 'spiritual healing'.

"Since 2003 I am on the spiritual path due to severe vision-problems (deterioration and detachment of retinas), which urged me to give up my career. I studied hundreds of spiritual books, I am initiated into Kriya-Yoga in the line of

Paramahamsa Yogananda and Roy Eugene Davis; I follow now a Taoist Buddhist path (Cosmic Freedom Qigong) to heal my eyes (trips to a healer in Brazil, John of God, helped me to avoid becoming totally blind. Now in one eye the retina is partially detached, with one eye I can see 30 %."

"No doctor can help me anymore. I already had 13 surgeries (both eyes, I think 10 in the left, 3 in the right eye). In both eyes the vitreous body has been removed, silicone has been filled into the eyeball (to re-attach the retina) and has then been removed again. In the left eye the procedure has been repeated without any success. In both eyes I have artificial lenses, because the operations had damaged the natural lens. There is no effective treatment with conventional medicine any more, it is over since 2003. I really did everything what was possible; during one of the operations there was a problem with local anaesthetics and I felt every stitch of a needle in my left eye. I got some treatments with eye-laser, the first of which was so painful that my whole body was wet with sweat after treatment. I was in hell. Only my trips to Brazil to "John of God" had helped me a bit – my eye doctor (an internationally well-known expert) was astonished that I had not become totally blind in both eyes. She even told me to go to Brazil again! In 2003 I had already purchased a gun to commit suicide, but after my first trip to Brazil (April 2004) my condition improved and again I hoped for a healing. In Brazil I was very brave: John of God claims to be a medium for high Beings (King Salomon, Ignatius from Loyola ...) who accomplishes spiritual operations through his body and I trusted him. I got a knife directly into the edge of my eyeball, hoping that his claims were true and they were. I had nothing to lose. There is no apparent other illness in my physical body, no diabetes, nothing. With healthy eyes I would be in a very, very good condition, apart from now being too fat out of frustration. This was ... the reason for the beginning of my spiritual quest. In my *case extraordinary spiritual power is necessary for my healing. New retina cells must be produced and the retina in the left eye must be re-attached... Currently I try again 'cellevelhealing'.* <u>*They had amazing results. I already got 3 treatments, two more are scheduled, [but] till now no result, let us see.*</u>"

The last sentence of this letter, underlined, already points to the Life-Medical 'diagnosis' that was arrived over seven months of correspondence with the patient. For though it begins with a claim that the healing method referred to by the patient had "amazing results", it concludes with a totally contradictory admission that "till now no result". The patient then adds "let us see" – but seems oddly *blind* to the contradiction, as if unwilling to face up to the fact or *see* that the method had not had the "amazing results" he wanted for himself.

I have italicised the word *'see'* both because of its relation to the patient's sight (which has since deteriorated by a further 10% in one eye) and also because of countless similar examples of statements made by the patient in the course of his correspondence with the Life Doctor – in all of which he appeared not to have understood or 'seen' what the Life Doctor had written to him – giving rise to the conclusion that he did not actually *want to see*. I should stress that the patient did not initially know about Life Doctoring or write to the Life Doctor as a *therapist* but rather as a spiritual teacher and *yogin* – someone who the patient believed could either heal him instantly or help him to develop extraordinary yogic powers with which to miraculously heal himself.

As a result, most of the patient's initial correspondence was *very narrowly focussed* on questions relating to detailed terminological and 'technical' aspects of yogic practice. Here again I emphasise the term *narrowly focused* – with its optical and visual connotations. Indeed, on many occasions the Life Doctor deliberately opted for *visual metaphors* in his correspondence with the patient in order to emphasise their significance for his sight problems and even pointing out to him that he had done so – by referring for example to *blindspots* in his thinking. Over the course of the correspondence however, what became ever more clear was the patient's fundamental unwillingness to *see* yoga and meditation as a method of attaining profound *insight* into himself and into his own medical condition – rather than as offering a mere method or set of theories and techniques for attaining miraculous powers of self-healing.

Below are just a few examples of language used by the patient in his emails which show instead how *fixated* his spiritual 'vision' was on transcending his body and on using spiritual powers and his 'third eye' to instantaneously and miraculously "burn away" his condition rather than gain any *insight* into it – let alone that of any other human beings:

"It must be possible to bring divine perfection to the physical plane."

"It must be possible to heal instantaneously by yogic powers."

"I clearly refer to what is called 'a miracle' by ordinary human beings."

"I want to be physically strong and healthy like a ferocious tiger, a mental genius and a spiritual giant with remarkable powers."

On the other hand, he admits that *"it was always a struggle for me to meditate"* and that *"to identify with another human being is for me quite terrifying ... my own weaknesses are enough."*

Though right from the start of correspondence with the patient, it was recommended that he read materials on Life Doctoring, and ask himself the sorts of question a Life Doctor would do, he did not initially do so. And even when the basic principles of Life Medicine were shared with him through correspondence, the patient – like many in search of spiritual 'healing' – had great difficulty in truly 'seeing', let alone heeding the basic idea that a specific illness might hold a specific meaning for the individual, that this meaning might itself be something worthy of *meditating* upon – and that in this way his illness might itself have a spiritual message for him and come to serve as his principal spiritual teacher and healer.

Indeed it seemed at times that this particular patient's 'reading' of the Life Doctor's letters was highly selective – as if he often did not even *optically register* those parts of them dealing with the nature and meaning of illness – let alone take any interest in the suggestion that a particular illness is always *chosen* by the individual for a well-intentioned reason and that its history must be viewed in the larger context of the patient's life story, life world and relationships.

On the contrary, it became ever more clear that this patient's vision of attaining healing powers over his illness *and* the very sight problems he sought to heal were both in fact *symptoms* – symptoms made particularly *visible* through his written correspondence – in which he continued to show little understanding or interest in any form of 'enlightenment' based on illuminating and meditative *in-sight*. And even without any experience of it he adopted a stereotypical negative viewpoint that any form of insight-based counselling was merely 'dredging the mud'.

Given that this was a patient, who, despite his serious sight problems simply 'did not want to see' the point of Life Doctoring, the Life Doctor felt that all he could do was to share with the patient precisely this Life-Medical insight – which itself had all to do *with* the patient's lacking interest in and capacity for deep 'in-sight' into himself and others.

Below I cite from two emails that constituted part of the climax of the Life Doctor's attempt to get the patient to 'see' the meaning of Life Medicine and the potential benefits of Life Doctoring, albeit taking care to do so in a way that respected the patient's relationship to him as 'spiritual teacher':

"All that you write confirms to me there may indeed be an important role that Life Doctoring can play in your life – though in a way very different from seeking a spiritual or biological 'miracle' cure of any sort. For I see your spiritual search for a miracle cure as more of a hindrance than a help.

The reason is that every healer you have been too, and every form of healing you have tried in order to find a cure for your eye condition is essentially a denial that it has any meaning. It seems that for you, as well as for the doctors and healers you have gone to, the only 'meaning' of your illness and what it can teach you seems to lie in finding a way to get rid of it.

But think of it this way: if your illness wants to be your most intimate and important spiritual teacher but all you want to learn from it is how to annihilate that illness – then you are looking for ways to annihilate your own teacher - in fact trying to kill it!

If and when you are ready to accept that this might be the most basic and important in-sight I can give you, then we can begin to consider ways and means in which, with my help – and through the reading and writing you are still (miraculously!) able to do - Life Medicine and Life Doctoring might bring you to a different and to a healing understanding of what your illness might be seeking to teach you.

From the point of view of Life Medicine 'the illness is the cure'. Life Doctoring is about finding out what the illness is attempting to cure in the patient!!!"

A short response to this message was then received from the patient in which he stated:

"... I really do not know what it is that I do not want to see. I will meditate that."

Since the Life Doctor's own email had already indicated to the patient what it was he did not want to see, a second e-mail was sent under the subject header 'What I see you as not seeing...' - once again making this as explicit as possible in the hope that this time the patient would 'see it'.

Your questions and vision have always been very <u>narrowly focussed</u> on 'techniques' of meditation. Throughout our *correspondence however, I have tried to encourage an insight-based approach to your questions rather than a purely detached and technique-based one. I believe cultivating such an insight-based approach to life is also of central importance in relation to your eye problems.*

You write that you "do not know what it is that I do not want to see".

So how about looking inside??!! And also listening inside and feeling inside.

That way you can come to your own answers – your own insights.

That is why I believe it terribly important that you learn to understand 'meditation' in a new way – not just as a set of techniques but as taking time to look inside yourself - for insights that can arise from feeling awareness.

Unless you learn to value deep personal and philosophical insights much more than you value yogic techniques and powers, and unless you learn to look inside yourself to feel for and find such insights, then I fear your eyes will just force you to do so.

For through increasing loss of 'out-sight' or even blindness you may eventually be unable to do anything <u>but</u> 'look inside' and also <u>listen</u> more deeply to yourself and others.

Put simply, through the decrease in your vision I believe <u>your eyes themselves</u> are telling you what you don't see – namely that despite all your knowledge and will power, without valuing and cultivating feeling in-sight, but instead continuing to narrow your thinking and spiritual vision either to detached intellectual and theoretical knowledge or to mastering yogic powers and *techniques to exercise in a detached way over your body, then your inner self or Atman will continue to narrow the vision of one or both of your bodily eyes through retinal detachment and eventually cut off your 'out-sight' completely. In other words, your illness - as your spiritual teacher - is saying that if you refuse to see inside you will lose your outer sight. It is therefore also urging you to put all your efforts into <u>seeing the difference</u> - perhaps for the first time in your life - between knowledge and wisdom, between your detached intellect and theoretical knowledge and deep feeling insight into yourself - and between manipulative techniques on the one hand and basic inner truths on the other. Using theoretical knowledge to attain power <u>over</u> your body from a detached ego or I are no substitute for your body's own inner knowing and powers of healing – and certainly no remedy for a detached retina in your eye – a clear symbol of your own detachment from yourself and others.*

The only substantive response to the message of these letters – and to an accompanying request for them to be incorporated into a case example in this book – was puzzlement that the author should wish to present a case study in which the patient had not been healed. This of course, simply re-affirmed the patient's misunderstanding of Life Medicine and Life Doctoring as an approach to medicine whose validity could only be proven by its effectiveness in healing the patient's illness – rather than offering potentially *life-transforming* and *healing understandings* of and insights into that illness. As for the idea that an illness might be there to *heal and transform the patient* – it was, again, simply not seen or registered on the mental *retina* of this patient – 'the man who did not want to see'.

PART 5
ON LIFE DOCTORING

What is Life Doctoring?

LIFE DOCTORING is therapeutic counselling for serious or chronic illness. It is about 'treating the patient and not the illness' – by exploring links between illness and life – in particular the relation between the emergence of symptoms and significant life changes.

"It is changes that are chiefly responsible for disease." Hippocrates

What is a Life Doctor?

A Life Doctor is a psychotherapist trained in Life Medicine and able to provide Life Doctoring for symptoms of all sorts, both 'mental' and 'physical'.

A Life Doctor is not a conventionally trained biomedical doctor and is not qualified to prescribe any form of conventional medical treatment.

Yet a Life Doctor is not only a medically well-informed counsellor and consultant, but also possesses different types of medical knowledge and understanding of a sort that ordinary doctors do not receive in their training.

The Life Doctor will never seek to prevent a patient seeing or seeking advice from an ordinary doctor or medical specialist, but will instead explore the patient's experience of orthodox medical practice and practitioners and the meaning this experience holds for them.

The Life Doctor however, will ask questions of a sort very different to those put by ordinary doctors or specialist consultants – whose main role is to come to a biomedical 'diagnosis' of a patient's symptoms and to offer corresponding forms of treatment.

The Life Doctor will also advise the patient about the possible dangers and/or side effects of different forms of biomedical testing and treatment.

What Life Doctoring offers:

Opportunities for you to share your personal experience of illness and of medical services and treatments with a knowledgeable and informed counsellor independent of the medical profession.

Quality listening time – and a different type of listening – of a sort that doctors and consultants have no time for.

Healing of a sort that can only begin with being fully *heard* as an individual *human being* – not reduced to a 'case' of some hypothetical 'disease'.

Advice in making informed choices about medical tests and treatments, including their potential dangers and side-effects.

Help in revealing the true story of your illness – its biographical as well as 'medical' history – as well as its impact on your current life.

Awareness of possible relational dimensions of your illness – its connection to your personal, family and social relationships, past and present.

The chance to discover significant links between your illness on the one hand and significant changes and events in your past or present life on the other.

Ways to put you more in touch with your body and what it may be telling you – or seeking to tell others.

Greater trust in your body's own knowing as opposed to any body of medical beliefs.

Help in bringing to light the questions your illness may itself be there to make you ask yourself about your life.

Help in understanding and relating to your illness in ways free of the fears that diagnostic labels so often arouse.

New forms of healing based on meditating our bodies rather than medicating them.

Important knowledge, advice and support in preparing for consultations with doctors, consultants, surgeons or other health professionals.

Prevention from getting entrapped by standard medical or psychiatric procedures - being reduced to a mere 'case' of some clinically diagnosed disease.

Protection from being persuaded into accepting potentially dangerous, counter-productive or even life-threatening forms of orthodox bio-medical testing and treatment.

The Practice of Life Doctoring (1)

Life Doctoring is therapy for serious and chronic illness. Its focus however, is on the patient's felt or lived body and not just on the clinical body or the body seen merely as a complex biological machine. The Life Doctor understands the body not as a biological machine but as a living biological language of the human being and symptoms of illness as the 'speech' or expression of the patient's life situation, life world and life history as a whole. The practical starting point of Life Doctoring is therefore precisely the type of questions that most doctors tend not to ask (see page 50). These relate to what was going on in the patient's life preceding the onset of symptoms, what they stop or hinder the patient from doing, the thoughts and feelings that accompany their symptoms and how they make the patient feel – that is to say, in what way they alter the patient's very sense of self – their body identity. At the same time, like any doctor, the Life Doctor must take a complete medical history of the patient – including all forms of testing and treatment they have undergone, what they have been led to believe about their condition and their experience of how they have been handled by doctors and other medical professionals.

The Life Doctor must also be capable of in-depth research and understanding of purely biological and biomedical understandings of the patient's condition. Like the General Practitioner, the Life Doctor is essentially a 'generalist' and not a specialist in these conditions. What distinguishes the Life Doctor however, is their capacity to 'read' even the most detailed biological and biomedical accounts of the nature and 'causes' of an illness in a very different way from that of a biomedical physician. For often the very language and terminology used in biological medicine itself, and the biological processes they are used to describe, can themselves be highly *symbolic.* This applies even to the very *names* given to certain conditions – for example the diagnostic term *lupus erythematosus* – meaning 'red wolf' and associated with dermatological symptoms such as red patches on the skin.

"Systemic lupus erythematosus ... often abbreviated to SLE or lupus, is a systemic autoimmune disease (or autoimmune connective tissue disease) that can affect any part of the body. As occurs in other autoimmune diseases, the immune system attacks the body's cells and tissue, resulting in inflammation and tissue damage. It is a Type III hypersensitivity reaction caused by antibody-immune complex formation. The course of the disease is unpredictable, with periods of illness (called *flares*) alternating with remissions. The disease occurs nine times more often in women than in men, especially in women in child-bearing years ages 15 to 35, and is also more common in those of non-European descent."

Wikipedia

Case Example 5

The patient in question first began to experience symptoms of lupus after coming off a treatment course of anti-depressants which lasted many years. The depression had followed the death of her grandmother, with whom she had a highly ambivalent relation. The symptoms of lupus had recently 'flared' again when it became a matter of financial importance to consider selling her mother's house – which she now occupied together with her partner but which the grandmother – a family matriarch – had insisted should always remain in the family.

As a woman, the patient felt responsible and sympathetic to the idea of maintaining a matriarchal line. On the other hand, she harboured deep feelings of anger at the way her mother had always been treated by the grandmother. These unexpressed feelings of anger and rage prevented her from, in any way, mourning the death of the grandmother and led instead to years of affect-less depression – the lack of affect being intensified by the anti-depressants themselves. Even after coming off them however, the patient's anger itself had never been given an opportunity to fully 'flare up'.

In consultations with the Life Doctor the patient gave a consistent impression of meek submissiveness – a strong parallel to her mother's submissive position in relation to the grandmother. At the same time the patient also experienced a sense of guilt at the idea of selling the house passed down by her grandmother. For to do so would be a betrayal, not just of the grandmother herself, but of the patient's own 'feminism', which had long found expression in an interest in Wiccan and other pagan forms of religiosity involving worship of the feminine aspect of divinity (which is sometimes called the 'great mother' – itself another term for 'grandmother').

The Life Doctor's analysis of the patient's illness in the context of her life history was that it was essentially rooted in a conflicted 'love-hate' relationship to her grandmother. On the one hand, she identified with what the grandmother symbolised for her (identification being an essential element of 'love') whilst on the other hand hating her for the way she had aggressively mistreated her own mother and reduced her to a state of passive servility. This is where the medical terminology itself revealed a new symbolic layer. For from the perspective of Life Medicine, auto-immune disorders – in which the body attacks itself – are an expression of guilt. The patient *punishes* themselves physiologically for feelings of guilt by directing the anger behind this guilt inwardly (through the body seeing its own cells as foreign or 'non-self') rather than this anger being consciously directed outwardly towards its true object – in this case the patient's grandmother.

"There are several explanations ventured for the term *lupus erythematosus*. *Lupus* is Latin for wolf, and *erythro* is derived from ερυθρός, Greek for 'red'. All explanations originate with the reddish, butterfly-shaped malar rash that the disease classically exhibits across the nose and cheeks.

1. In various accounts, some doctors thought the rash resembled the pattern of fur on a wolf's face.

2. In other accounts, doctors thought that the rash, which was often more severe in earlier centuries, created lesions that resembled wolf bites or scratches.

3. Another account claims that the term "lupus" did not come from Latin directly, but from the term for a French style of mask that women reportedly wore to conceal the rash on their faces. The mask is called a 'loup', French for 'wolf'."

Anger and rage are of course associated with the colour red – and for a biomedical diagnosis of *lupus erythematosus* (red wolf) the appearance of thick red patches or blisters on the skin is highly significant. So much for the 'red' in 'red wolf' but what about the wolf – itself an aggressive and predatory creature. The Life Doctor's interpretation of the patient's illness came to clearest expression through an intuitive link between the biomedical name and nature of her illness, her life history – and their common relation to the story of 'Little Red Riding Hood'. To the Life Doctor the patient appeared as 'Little Red Riding Hood'. The question was then – who 'ate' her grandmother? Clearly not a wolf, but perhaps someone who felt aggressive 'h-ate' for her i.e. a part of the patient herself. The patient's inability to mourn her grandmother's death might also therefore have been due to her feeling that her own suppressed feelings of hate were what killed her grandmother, thus compounding the patient's guilt. In a nutshell then, the patient developed symptoms of the illness known as 'red wolf' by virtue of never allowing herself to affirm, identify with and live out – what the wolf in the story symbolised – not just her blood-red anger towards the grandmother but the aggressive side of herself as a whole.

The key question for the Life Doctor then, was not how to 'treat' or 'cure' the lupus (it is regarded even in biomedicine as incurable) but rather an entirely different *type* of question. This was the question of what the illness was seeking to cure in the patient – in what way it was seeking to transform her? In the context of her particular history and the Red Riding Hood fable, it seems this question could be put more specifically: in what ways, besides 'flares' of her symptoms and bodily inflammations, did or did not the patient grant herself permission to consciously get 'inflamed' or 'flare up' with anger – and to fully feel, embody and show the true face of this anger? For this would allow herself to live out the 'red wolf' within her – rather than playing the role of 'little red riding hood' in relation to that wolf.

The personal significance of the fable for this patient lay in the way that the wolf symbolised *both* the aggressive side of her grandmother and the patient's own feelings of anger toward her. In a sense it could be said that the patient, like her mother, had quite simply 'swallowed' her grandmother – not in a consciously predatory, hostile or aggressive way but by simply internalising or taking the grandmother inside herself – where she became the object of chronic or recurrent auto-immune attacks by her own body – which simply embodied the patient's dual and conflicted relation to the grandmother – both identifying with her as a part of herself and at the same time dis-identifying with her – leading the body to identify and attack her own cells as if they were 'foreign' or 'non-self' bodies.

The unconscious, internal and biologically routed attack on her grandmother no doubt further exacerbated the patient's chronic psychological guilt – thus creating a vicious cycle which maintained the symptoms of lupus – chronically recurrent symptoms.

The bodily symptoms themselves also corresponded to a specific state of consciousness characterised by a felt sense of weakness and therefore in themselves symbolised a type of recurrent submission *to* the grandmother – even whilst biologically symbolising an attempt to dis-identify from her on a cellular level – thus rendering her own cells subject to auto-immune 'attack'.

Yet, as mentioned, the patient came to the Life Doctor in a specific life situation in which her guilt – and the aggressive anger behind it – were exacerbated by the conflict she felt at perhaps having to sell her grandmother's house, this exacerbation leading to what biomedicine itself terms a 'flare' of the lupus. Biomedicine seeks causes for such flares in so-called 'environmental triggers' such as allergens, bacteria or viruses. Yet in this way the 'environment' in question is in no way connected with the patient's life world – their social and relational environment as a *human being* - but instead reduced to a possible source of infections or inflammations affecting the human body. Life Medicine, on the other hand, understands 'environmental triggers' as having *essentially* to do with particular events in the patient's social and relational environment – precisely because it is emotional triggers coming from this environment that may render an individual more *susceptible* to 'environmental triggers' in the purely biomedical sense.

Biomedical treatment of lupus symptoms takes the form of both anti-malarial and so-called 'anti-inflammatory' or 'immuno-suppressant' drugs. Both are an attempt to render the patient's body biologically *incapable* of expressing – through auto-immune responses and bodily inflammation – deeply buried and inflamed *feelings* which, in the absence of direct vocal, emotional or behavioural expression, will naturally seek a way of 'flaring up' and of literally 'coming to the surface' through *skin* inflammations. Yet if prevented from doing so by biomedical drugs, the danger is that the 'inflammation' will progressively begin to damage internal organs too – thus distracting the focus of both doctor and patient even further from the *basic question* of what the illness is there to 'cure' in the patient i.e. what understandings it is offering the patient and how it is seeking to change the patient in a way that would allow them to embody and express their dis-ease in a way other than through bodily illness and its symptoms.

Here again we come to the central question of Life Medicine, both in general and as exemplified in particular through so-called 'auto-immune' disorders – namely the potential role of the Life Doctor in acting as a midwife in helping patients feel and give birth to a new bodily *sense of self* or 'body identity' – as opposed to remaining stuck with an over-rigid or internally conflicted body identity that finds expression only biologically and through illness symptoms. In the specific case of the patient referred to here, she came to recognise that the key to turning her illness into a cure lay in finding ways to overcome weak and submissive sides of her identity and instead to embody her anger and rage in ways that avoided the need for aggressive flares of her symptoms – flares which were also accompanied by periods of severe physical weakness. Here she was helped by some of the principal non-verbal methods of Life Doctoring explained and described in more detail in the following chapter on the Practice of Life Doctoring.

In this case the patient was asked to simply feel in her body and show the Life Doctor – silently and face to face – the true *face* of her feelings; both her un-mourned feelings of sadness but also her *anger* in relation to her grandmother (or to anyone). The exercise proved strongly cathartic for the patient in first surrendering to her sense of sadness and weakness and then feeling and showing the face of her anger. This was not a face marred by the red patch symptomatic of *lupus* but did indeed have qualities of aggressive fierceness of a *wolf-like* character – as opposed to the patient's previously *pale-faced* expression and submissive or compliant demeanour. The patient also understood the difference between allowing herself occasional emotional flares or verbal 'outbursts' of anger on the one hand, and, on the other hand using continued practice of the exercises she had been taught to silently *body* that anger through her facial expression and the look in her eyes – knowing from experience that in this way she could be coming to embody a new, less weak, sad or submissive sense of self, feeling it pervading her felt body and transforming her body identity as a whole. It should be emphasised here that in dealing with long-term or chronic conditions, long-term practice of exercises introduced by the Life Doctor are of no less importance than the healing insights and understandings that Life Medicine offers.

The practice of Life Doctoring however, always begins with a search for the 'hidden story' behind a patient's illness in the form of what is called a 'pathobiography'. And indeed psychoanalysts such as Luis Chiozza have evolved a specific form of medical practice which they call 'the pathobiographical method'. This involves gathering a detailed biography of the patient which is then analysed by a team which includes not only psychoanalysts but also physicians and biomedical specialists. One important difference between Chiozza's method and the practice of Life Doctoring however, lies in the fact that the latter does not rely on any form of elaborate psychoanalytic theory or esoteric terminology to 'interpret' the symbolism of a patient's illness. Instead it attends purely and simply to what Freud called 'organ speech', and in particular to four distinct ways in which this finds expression:

1. In the language of biomedicine itself – for example by re-linking the purely medical meaning of terms such as 'inflammation' or 'flare' to their use in describing emotional states ('flaring up' or 'feeling inflamed' with anger).

2. In the physiological symptoms, functions and processes described in the language of bio-medicine (for example the language of immunology and of auto-immune disorders).

3. In the individual patient's lived experience of specific symptoms – as described in their own speech and as an expression of their lived or felt body.

4. Through the ways in which the specific life story and context of an individual patient's illness and its symptoms lends them a highly *individual* meaning.

In the past, and still in the work of Chiozza himself, psychoanalytic medicine has tended to seek 'standard' analyses of particular illnesses. This is not to say that there are no general understandings that can be drawn about the life meaning of particular organic disorders or dysfunctions – but this can be done only through Life Doctoring i.e. through exploration of highly *individual* cases of them. Life Medicine then, is not just a set of fixed general principles to be applied in and to particular 'cases' but is an expanding body of medical knowledge drawn from the very practice of these principles through 'Life Doctoring' – which serves also as a form of *on-going research* into the relation between language, life and illness.

The Practice of Life Doctoring (2)

As a practice, Life Doctoring is not simply a type of counselling or analytic 'talking cure'. That is because its principal focus is not on the causes and 'cures' but on the *meaning* of a specific illness and specific symptoms for the individual patient. Just as importantly however, as a form of therapy its principal 'instrument' is not just a new body of intellectual knowledge and insights but – no less importantly – the Life Doctor's own inwardly felt body. For it is only through this that the Life Doctor can come to *directly* sense and resonate with the underlying *dis-ease* that pervades the patient's own inwardly felt body i.e. their own 'lived body'. Cultivating the capacity to sense the felt inwardness of a patient's body takes us to a level much deeper than intellectual insight or emotional empathy alone. For the individual's lived body is essentially not a fleshly body of tissue and organs but the body of their own feeling awareness of themselves, other people and the world around them. As such it is made up of particular tones, textures and tissues *of* awareness – each with their own basic tones of awareness or 'feeling tones'. Like audible *vocal or musical tones* these silent feeling tones or tonalities of awareness have their own distinctive qualities such as tonal pitch and tone 'colour', brightness or darkness, warmth or coolness, lightness or heaviness, flatness or sharpness, softness or hardness, clarity or dullness, hollowness or resonance, harmony or dissonance. They are not just echoed in vocal and music tones but also embodied in cellular, organic tone and muscular tone. Felt tonalities of awareness or feeling tones are what not only tone and colour our moods but also determine, in a quite literal sense, the 'sound-ness' of our health.

Particular 'elemental' *qualities* of feeling tone however – qualities such as fiery vitality, airy spaciousness, watery fluidity or earthly solidity may be more or less dominant or lacking. Thus, in the previous case example, the Life Doctor sensed a deep quality of warmth but a far lesser degree of both fieriness and solidity in the patient's overall feeling tone –– an absence echoed also in the corresponding qualities of the patient's tone of voice. Part of the therapy also consisted of 'voice training' – teaching the patient to introduce a greater solidity, strength, amplitude and quality of fiery vitality to her voice tone. This was not done though any standard methods of 'voice coaching' but through first attuning her to particular qualities of her own inwardly heard speech – her 'inner voice' and its tones - and then imparting these tones of her inner voice with particular qualities of feeling tone, volume, fullness etc – all *before* vocalising them audibly.

This particular method of Life Doctoring is one of many designed to *amplify* the patient's awareness of silent inner tones of feeling precisely *by* giving them outer expression – whether through the vocal organs and vocal tones or silently, through their face and eyes. The basic methodological principle at the root of all these practices is the principle of 'morphic resonance', a term coined by Rupert Sheldrake but which Life Medicine understands in a very specific way – namely that giving expressive outer form (*morphe*) to particular feeling tones (in particular through the voice, face and the look in our eyes) we both *amplify* and bring ourselves into greater *resonance* with these feeling tones – and thereby with our lived body as such. This in turn allows us to learn to consciously modulate our overall mood or tone of feeling in a similar way that we modulate our tone of voice – by first sensing the tones we wish to make audible as silent tones of feeling.

From the perspective of Life Medicine, the individual's visible body speech (silent and vocal) is a further and fundamental dimension of what Freud called 'organ speech' - for it can be used to give form to, amplify and/or add to a patient's awareness of otherwise weaker or wholly unfelt dimensions and qualities of their feeling awareness and *its* body – the lived body. :

"The outer shape of a person reflects his inner mood. Changing that shape can change his mood."

David Boadella

Here 'shape' can refer to anything from a particular posture, tilt of the head, look in the eyes or indeed the smallest feature of a person's facial expression and the look in their eyes.

"Consciousness in another's face. Look into someone else's face, and see the consciousness in it, and a particular shade of consciousness."

Ludwig Wittgenstein

Perhaps *the* single most innovative and advanced method of Life Doctoring – and one that requires much training is practiced through extended, close-up eye contact with the patient. Here the Life Doctor uses the motility and expressiveness of his or her own face and eyes to seek for and precisely *mirror* particular features that he sees and senses in the patient's face and their eyes – features that no matter how subtle or fleeting can be seen and felt to give expression to deep and deeply significant feeling tones.

Through this very precise *art* of facial and ocular mirroring the Life Doctor can:

1. *Attune* to particular tones and qualities of feeling in the patient by consciously observing and intentionally mirroring them back to the patient.
2. *Amplify* both their own and the patient's lived experience of these tones and qualities of feeling – thus bringing the patient into greater contact with them.
3. *Transform* the patient's experience of these tones and qualities of feeling, in particular by moving from a stage of mirroring the patient's 'emotional' feelings to mirroring these back purely *as* tones of feeling – comparable to purely musical tones and their sensuous qualities.

This three-stage method of Life Doctoring I call 'Transformative Resonance'.

In the previous case example, it was applied by the Life Doctor in roughly the following way:

1. Mirroring back in an intentionally amplified and intensified way a surface look of resignation, surrender and 'sadness' in the patient's face and eyes.

2. Mirroring back in an intentionally amplified and intensified way glimpses of the weakly felt 'anger' latent within that sadness.

3. Mirroring this 'anger' in a transformed way i.e. not merely as an 'emotional' feeling but as a purely *sensuous* feeling of power, strength and fiery vitality arising from the very core of the patient's being.

4. Consciously and intentionally *imparting* to the patient's lived body the Doctor's own bodily sense of the patient's elemental 'core' of fiery vitality, strength and potency.

The recognition of the importance of the face and eyes in all forms of therapy is not new. And it must therefore play a central role in any form of therapy in which the therapist takes the client seriously as 'some-body' – not just a 'talking head'. Mirroring a patient's facial expression and the look in their eyes facilitates a process of mimesis which is central to sensing, attuning to and resonating with the patient's lived body as a whole.

"Without ... willingness to read the secret expression and to nurse it into life, any therapeutic encounter is gravely weakened."

"Facing is concerned with recognition, with how we see people, with the qualities of lumination that develop when people really face each other and with the forms of illumination that flash out of such contact. Insight develops in step with outlook.

If a person can let his inner self be seen by another, he begins to become recognisable to himself and can then look within, not in the sense of any sterile introspection, but in the sense of learning to love and accept who he is, and so recognise himself." David Boadella, *Lifestreams*

Boadella also quotes an account of Wilhelm Reich's work with a patient who suddenly began "seeing the world with new eyes", the fear and hate having gone out of them. As a result he also saw his therapist differently. The process began with Reich noticing a new gleam in the patient's eyes, which...

" .... together with the shifting of the eyes and head, had brought up a new expression out of the depths of his eyes and being. It was a flirtatious, come-hither look, a sort of wink, with a raising of the eyelids, eyebrows and forehead and a moving of the eyeballs to one side, accompanied by a suggestive tilting of the head, in the same direction. As the therapist began to imitate this expression and the patient began to make better contact with it, the whole face participated in it, at first with a blushing shame-facedness, and then to the tune of a hearty laugh." (ibid)

Reich did not merely "face" or "confront" the patient with a *verbal* mirror or interpretation of what he had seen and felt in the face and eyes of the patient but used his own body to mirror it back directly - thus helping the patient to feel it more fully. As a result a "miracle" happens:

"Suddenly the patient was startled and opened his eyes wide with astonishment. While he was looking at the therapist the latter's face had suddenly become soft, and glowed with light...He saw the world differently, as a good and pleasurable place to be in and as a future place of 'heaven' and not the 'hell' it had been before." (ibid)

Bodily sensing and identification is involved even in the understanding of verbal and indeed philosophical thinking itself. Wittgenstein again:

"I begin to understand a philosophy by feeling my way into its existential manner, by reproducing the tone and accent of the philosopher."

The Life Doctor must be trained in many highly subtle and multi-faceted arts or 'yogas' of bodily sensing and residence – all based on the principle of Morphic Resonance and the practice of Transformative Resonance. Through acute sensitivity not just to the patient's voice, but to the very tone of their words and language itself – and through practicing a subtle and sophisticated 'yoga of the face or eyes' through mirroring and 'transformative resonance' – the Life Doctor can learn to both see and feel their way into the lived body of the client – quite literally experiencing the eyes as 'windows of the soul' and both the patient's face and the look in their eyes as the expression of a particular 'shade of consciousness' or feeling tone.

It is in this way that the Life Doctor can gain a tangible sense of those tones and qualities of feeling *not* fully embodied by the patient, but instead 'somatised' – given symbolic expression through their symptoms or organic illness.

"Every feeling is an embodiment attuned in this or that way, a mood that bodies in this or that way."

Martin Heidegger

What distinguishes Life Medicine and its therapeutic methods from those of psychoanalysis is that psychoanalytic theory understands illness symptoms only as symbolic 'somatisations' of feelings that the patient is not capable of signifying through *verbal* speech or symbolising through mental and dream imagery. 'Somatisation', in other words, is understood solely as a failure to give expression to unconscious feeling in words – hence the emphasis of psychoanalysis on verbalisation and verbal interpretations of the symbolism of dreams and mental images.

In contrast, Life Doctoring understands 'somatisation' as a failure to find ways to consciously *embody* feelings through the patient's overall body language and speech, of which verbal language speech is itself but one dimension. It is not just through some form of emotional illiteracy or 'alexithymia' as it is called, but also and above all through lacking a rich and expressive enough *body language* by which to 'speak' our feelings that what Freud called 'organ speech' is forced to take the form of illness symptoms or unconscious 'somatisation'.

It is not just that which we cannot express in words but above all that which we cannot expressively *embody* that we 'somatise'. Thus, referring back to our case example, it is not just someone who cannot articulate a feeling of anger in words but principally someone who cannot simply *show* anger through their body speech - their posture, face and eyes - who is in greater danger of turning that anger inwards or losing contact with it. Indeed someone may well be capable of verbally reporting a feeling of anger (or any emotion) without *fully* feeling it. For it is through expression in the 'shape' or form of their *body speech* that awareness of feelings (and of different tones *of* awareness or 'feeling tones') are not only given form but also *amplified* through resonance.

What is called 'emotional illiteracy' – to whatever degree it is evident and however important it is in itself – almost invariably *pales* in extent before the poverty of the average individual's body language and the limitations of their most basic 'alphabet' of postures, gestures, vocal tones, facial expressions and ways of communicating tones of feeling through the look in their eyes. This impoverishment of body speech and body language is in itself a form of generalised pathology – since it makes almost unavoidable the expression (*logos*) of a felt sense of dis-ease (*pathos*) through illness i.e. through 'pathological' bodily or behavioural symptoms.

Besides underlying moods or tones of feeling – or the absence thereof – the Life Doctor also uses their own lived body to sense five principal features of the lived body of the patient – its degree of motility, groundedness and centeredness, openness and boundedness.

That is why, in addition to 'pathobiographical' questioning (see *What Most doctors Don't Ask?*), seven *further* questions of a different sort are invariably put to the patient in the initial Life Doctoring consultations:

1. **To what degree, on a scale of 1 to 10, can you inwardly feel your body as a whole – from top to toe – including not just your head or upper body, but your entire lower body below the waist, including your legs and reaching down to the soles of your feet?**

2. To what extent, on a scale of 1 to 10, are you aware of the entire surface skin and musculature of your upper body – including the surface skin and musculature of your face and eyes, of the surface of your entire head – top, front, back and sides, and of your trunk – front, back and sides?

3. On an imaginary vertical line extending within you from the crown of your head to the soles of your feet, point to where you feel your *breathing* is centred.

4. On the same imaginary line point to where you feel your very *sense of self* is centred.

5. To what degree, on a scale of one to ten, do you feel yourself to be aware, not just of your body but of the entire space surrounding it in this room and all it contains?

6. Using your arms, indicate both the size of any clear and empty inner space or spaces you feel enclosed by your body and also *where* you feel that space or those spaces – whether just in your head, your upper body, or in your trunk as a whole including your abdomen. If you feel no clear and empty spaces at all within you, just say so.

7. Using both your arms to indicate a sphere or space around your body, show to what extent you feel yourself extending into space in a way that reaches *beyond the boundaries of your skin*.

The answers sensed and given to these questions tell the Life Doctor about the specific 'anatomy' of the patient's lived body, as well as providing suggestive keys to the patient about what it means to cultivate feeling awareness of their lived body as a whole – a body which is not enclosed or bounded by one's skin but embraces all the spaces within *and* around it. Such whole-body awareness is a foundation for well-being as well as for the patient's own capacity for self-doctoring.

The questions above also provide a foundation for teaching the patient to engage in four basic movements or motions of awareness that are central to both sustaining whole-body awareness. These basic motions of awareness are:

1. **Grounding** – recovering and sustaining whole-body awareness – in particular through heightened awareness of one's entire *lower body* below the waist as well as one's head and upper body.

2. **Centring** – learning to seat or centre both one's *breathing* and one's very *sense of self* within the lower abdomen – this being both the spiritual and physical centre of gravity of the human being i.e. the centre of both their lived body and their physical body.

3. **Opening** - using one's upper body surface to sense the entire space surrounding one's body as a whole and all other bodies within that space. In this way coming to experience one's entire body surface as 'all eye' and as a totally porous membrane – one through which one can experience oneself as literally *breathing in* one's *awareness* of the light and space around one.

4. **Facing** – giving form to a felt bodily sense of dis-ease through the look in one's face and eyes, thereby both intensifying that sense of dis-ease and also coming to feel it as an all-pervasive state of consciousness i.e. an underlying

mood, feeling tone or texture of awareness that can be actively bodied - rather than 'somatised' in the form of one or more localised bodily sensations or symptoms or organic disturbances.

Case Example 6

Patient: a 60 year old man teaching at a college and responsible also as a community elder for care and support of young people in difficulty.

Symptoms: heart arrhythmia, fainting spells, shortness of breath.

Biomedical diagnosis: atrial fibrillation (confirmed by ECG) and fibrosis of the lungs confirmed by X-ray - possibly connected through lack of sufficient oxygen and resultant shortness of breath.

Biomedical prognosis: possibility of early death (2-3 years) through progressive worsening of fibrosis in the lungs.

Medications prescribed: propranolol, badly tolerated because of side effects and replaced by sotalol – both intended to slow and regularise heart rate and reduce shortness of breath, Warfarin to reduce risk of stroke. Statins. Drugs to treat prostate enlargement.

Possible surgical interventions suggested:

- Heart surgery in the form of catheter ablation – used to destroy an area of the heart producing abnormal electrical circuits and resulting in disturbances of cardiac rhythm.

- Implantation of a pacemaker to regularise heartbeat.

Principle reasons for the patient arranging to see a Life Doctor:

- Concern about the prescribed medications and their actual or possible side effects.

- Dissatisfaction with what he experienced as a total lack of any expression of human warmth, empathy and interest on the part of the biomedical doctors and consultants he had seen (not one of them even asked him about his feelings regarding the possibility of death within 3 years).

- Intrinsic interest in the approach to illness represented by Life Medicine and Life Doctoring.

Initial questions presented by the Life Doctor:

Questions regarding the patient's life history, work and current relationship.

Questions concerning the exact life time and location, life context and situation in which the symptoms first occurred, and how the patient felt and responded to them.

Questions regarding the frequency and exact situations and locations in which the symptoms of atrial fibrillation tend to re-occur.

Initial impressions and information gained by the Life Doctor:

The patient was felt as a human being with deep and natural warmth and empathy, humour and interest in others as well as in philosophical issues surrounding both methods of counselling and therapy and medicine itself.

Elements emphasised by the patient in sharing his life history:

- Early experiences of abandonment. His father abandoned his mother and himself when he was three years old. His mother however, who suffered from on-going withdrawal symptoms resulting from long-term dependency on psychoactive prescription drugs (benzodiazepine 'tranquilisers') also abandoned him in a different way. This took the form of lack of attention, empathy or sustained listening. Her resulting and constant inner restlessness, anxiety, depression and self-preoccupation expressed itself in extreme impatience if, as a child, the patient did not instantaneously reply to her questions. Not being given even a moment's time for reflection and authentic self-expression induced a severe childhood stutter in the patient, since overcome.

- Abandonment by the mother of his children, leaving him in the position of sole carer for three young children without any social or familial support whatsoever even from his brother or sister. This was reinforced by his sister-in-law, who refused to allow visits or even telephone calls with his brother. It was during this period that the patient's symptoms emerged.

- In contrast, the patient frequently emphasised how much he enjoyed the human contact with his students and how much appreciation they expressed for his warmth, humanity and overall bearing towards them – for example the way he did not 'talk down' to them as a teacher, but, as well as offering valuable teaching and insights, also related to them as human beings in their own right in an authentic and non-formal or role-bound way.

Initial links made by the Life Doctor between the patient's illness and his life circumstances:

- Life history of abandonment and the responses to it resulting from the patient's symptoms.

- Notably, it was only *through* an initial severe bout of his symptoms while living as an isolated single father that, despite his sister-in-law's prohibitions, he took the decision to phone his brother and actively seek support.

- The patient's decision to write to and consult with the Life Doctor was made not just in the context of his medical diagnosis and prognosis, but also his experience (through his mother and others) of the potentially damaging effects of prescription drugs and his sense of not being treated as a human being by medical professionals. Proactively contacting the Life Doctor thus constituted a way in which the patient's *illness itself* led him to enact a healthy part of himself – one that refused to surrender to many life experiences of relational isolation and abandonment.

Other felt impressions from the initial consultation:

- The Life Doctor observed that at no point in the initial consultation did the patient say how his initial account of his illness and life, together with his current medical diagnosis and prognosis left him feeling or thinking (a question which no one, even his current partner, had at any time asked him). Instead the 'patient' simply took great pleasure and interest in the opportunity the consultation provided for warm, informal but also patient and therefore insight-generating communication provided by the Life Doctor himself - both as a human being and as a man of similar age with whom he shared common life values, understandings and even experiences.

- On the other hand, the Life Doctor felt, through the patient's downcast gaze and generally lowered lids, a bodily sense of something like an underlying mood of resignation behind the patient's otherwise animated, open and interest-full vocal communication. The mood of resignation seemed in contrast to the proactive and healthy steps taken by the patient in response to his experiences of abandonment that his symptoms had led him to enact - leading ultimately to the pleasure and interest he took in the Life-Doctoring consultation itself and his interest in having further sessions. At the same time, the Life Doctor observed that the patient was taking more of an interest in the consultation itself than in his own feelings about his illness. Together with the sensed mood of resignation, the Life Doctor became even more curious about what the essential existential or life 'dis-ease' of the patient might be, particularly since the patient had also reported an acute episode of his symptoms in which he felt he might be dying – but also felt quite happy to let go and resign himself to death - therefore in effect abandoning himself.

Between life and death - the patient's essential life dilemma:

Knowing something of the circumstances surrounding the emergence of the patient's symptoms – and knowing also that despite the fibrosis of his lungs and occasional shortness of breath walking up steep inclines, the patient was still able to take mile-long walks without any difficulty – the Life Doctor returned in the second session to the patient's symptoms of atrial fibrillation and asked the patient how frequently and in what particular circumstances he tended to experience them. The answer was quickly forthcoming and revealing – whenever he was at home with his current partner, towards whom he had long felt a loss of sexual attraction, who did not share any of his interests, with whom he could not discuss his work as a teacher or any deeper philosophical and life questions. Indeed it was his partner herself who - although the patient described her as very "loving and caring" – made clear that she felt abandoned by him merely by his reading a book in her presence. Lacking all forms of physical contact and sexual fulfilment from the patient led to a progressive increase in the weight gain that had first diminished his sexual desire for her since they met. However she was also limited in her willingness and capacity to openly discuss their physical relationship. This was made worse by personal and cross-cultural differences which made even attempts at mutual discussion of the future of their relationship very difficult.

Placed in the context of the patient's radically different experience of his world of work, the picture that emerged was one of the patient inhabiting two entirely separate and contrasting life worlds. One world was the spacious, enlivening, emotionally heartening, intellectually inspiring and also libidinally restorative (if not fulfilling) world of his close, authentic and heartfelt relationships with his students and co-teachers. This was a world in which he was able to embody his deepest values and abilities as a human being, share his greatest interests and at least feel if not fulfil strong sexual desires. The other world was the narrow, enclosed and stifling world of his sexually and communicatively unsatisfying home life and relationship with his partner. For this, in contrast, was a world he experienced each day as disheartening and deadening – in contrast to the enheartening and enlivening relational world of his work and students in which he also felt 'room to breathe'. It became clear to the Life Doctor that the bodily mood of resignation he had sensed in the patient had to do with the way the patient had resigned himself to living in these two contrasting worlds – one enlivening and enheartening, the other disheartening and deadening – leaving him with a life quite literally led 'between life and death'. The Life Doctor shared with the patient the direct parallels he saw between this, the essential 'dis-ease' of the patient, and his potentially life-threatening or life-shortening heart and lung symptoms and the 'disease' or 'disorders' by which they were biomedically labelled.

The patient's response to the life picture of his illness:

In the third session, the patient, when questioned, reported how much he had reflected on, understood and agreed with the 'life picture' of his illness offered by the Life Doctor at the end of the second session and how he also saw the clear relationship it revealed between his lung and heart condition and his current life situation. In this session too however, it also became clear to both doctor and patient that, in the context of his life picture of his illness, the biggest threat to the patient's health and life lay not in any biomedically labelled condition or prognosis but rather in resigning himself to a life led 'between life and death', i.e. between two life worlds, the one alive and the other dead. The Life Doctor suggested that the alternative to resignation or self-abandonment in this limbo state lay in understanding the lived dis-ease and its bodily symptoms as the expression and embodiment of a fundamental life dilemma – one which demanded careful consideration and perhaps new and courageous life decisions from him, not least with regards to his relationship to and sexual life with his current life partner – with whom it became clear again that he was extremely 'ill-at-ease'.

In this context the Life Doctor became aware, following this session, of a particular paradox of the patient's life dilemma and the potential life decisions it demanded from him – namely that were he to leave his relationship with his partner or pursue new relationships whilst staying within it, he himself would become the abandoner rather than the abandoned. On the other hand, it was already evident that he had for a long time inwardly been afraid of or abandoned all attempts to rescue or redeem the relationship, as had his partner herself – leaving it in a state of routinized, uncommunicative and death-like limbo, one in which they inhabited separate worlds even whilst living together.

It was agreed that future sessions would concentrate on the life dilemmas and decisions faced by the patient, together with (1) on-going monitoring of when, in what situations, to what degree and how often his symptoms occurred and (2) continued discussion of whether – or which – of the several different prescription drugs he was taking were necessary. Questions of the role and potential influence on health exerted by different beliefs about death – and the existence or not of an afterlife – were also placed on the agenda for further exploration.

Observation of the patient's mood and body language:

Last but not least, the Life Doctor felt a need to address what he felt as the patient's underlying mood of resignation in the face of his life circumstances and dilemmas. This was expressed very strongly in the patient's body language – in particular the tilt of his head and body, the look in his eyes and his facial expression as a whole. The Life Doctor observed that the patient tended almost invariably to tilt his head down to one side and towards his left shoulder. This was accompanied by a type of worried frown which drew his eyelids together almost completely – as if squinting in the face of a bright light – making eye contact with others impossible.

It was as if the patient had over the years got stuck in a habit of never fully 'holding his head high' rather than leaning it down to one side – and found it now extremely difficult to do so. His 'downcast gaze', in other words, had effectively become part of his body identity, as had his tendency not to open his eyes fully so that he could not 'look people straight in the eye.'

The Life Doctor responded to this by feeding back his observations of the patient's body language, mirroring them and explaining to him the principle that: *"The outer shape of a person reflects his inner mood"* (Boadella) and that *"Changing that shape can change his mood."*. Noting how even in close up eye contact with the patient – and despite attempts to straighten his head and neck – the patient still invariably held his head slightly tilted to one side, the Life Doctor gave the patient inter-session 'body homework'. This took the form of suggesting that he attempt to keep his head perfectly balanced and upright for an entire day or week – and to then see and feel how 'changing his shape' in this way and also looking people 'straight in the eye' might affect his bodily sense of self and alter both his mood of resignation and resigned mode of relating. For his current posture both embodied and reinforced these – not just in his relation to his partner but also his supervising manager.

Progression and Outcomes of the Life Doctoring Sessions:

The possibility of a less resigned and more proactive mode of relating – both verbally and bodily – was heeded by the patient with good results – initially however only in the context of his relationship to his supervisor, which he approached in a new, courageous and effective way.

Though he also made attempts to move closer to his partner, these were clearly not successful, and yet they gave further insight into his heart symptoms. For on further questioning he reported that his symptoms of atrial fibrillation started or became particularly acute not just in the presence of his partner but *specifically* on occasions when she indicated a desire for sex. The patient described how on such occasions he experienced strong inner feelings of guilt at not being able to *reciprocate* in any way the love and care he felt he received from her. Rather than openly and proactively sharing these feelings of guilt with her – which would itself have at least been a token of his reciprocal care for her – he would simply say he was "not in the mood", hiding both his feelings and the episodes of atrial fibrillation that accompanied them. And though the patient took on board a suggestion to make time to honestly share his feelings with his partner – and his reasons for not wanting sex – he found this extremely difficult to do . He even found it impossible to offer his partner any form of affectionate non-sexual contact such as a hug. Recognising that in this way he was effectively 'abandoning' his partner, The Life Doctor suggested that this might be a way of acting out his own history of abandonment by others as well as being part of his general and long-term inability to experience intimate connection with women except through sexual arousal and intercourse.

With regards to the patient's other symptom – shortness of breath – its initial diagnosis and prognosis through X-ray scans as a specific form of fibrosis of the lungs, one which might progressively worsen and even shorten his remaining life span to two years, was brought into question. For when the patient met his medical consultant again and asked why a decision had been taken *not* to conduct any further scans but instead to just regularly monitor the patient's lung function capacity, the consultant effectively admitted that the initial scan was not conclusive.

As a result, the patient reported having no more worries at all about having a potentially terminal illness – since it was the seemingly premature *medical diagnosis and prognosis* itself that had really 'taken his breath away' – causing more anxiety than his shortness of breath itself. And in the course of his sessions with the Life Doctor these had become and remained so mild as to be hardly even abnormal. The patient instead reported going on long walks again – for him both a major source of pleasure in life and also his means, besides teaching, of enjoying a sense of friendship and non-sexual bonding and connection with others.

This is not to imply that the sessions of Life Doctoring constituted, in and of themselves, a 'cure' for the patient's illnesses, but rather an opportunity to let them serve as a cure for the patient – firstly by showing how they expressed important aspects and dilemmas connected with past and current life and relationships, and also by urging him to find a new body identity – one in which a basic mood of resignation to life could be transformed, quite literally, by learning to 'hold his head high' and 'look people firmly in the eye'.

What can I do if I am a Biomedical Doctor?

Study more of the literature on Phenomenological, Existential and Psychoanalytic Medicine (See the list of 'Further Reading'.)

If you are in private practice, consider extending at least your initial consultations with each patient to up to an hour – to allow time to gather more information about their lives, life world and life history.

If you are working as a GP in the public health system:

Ask more questions about the patient's life and not just the symptoms they present with.

In particular, take opportunities to ask questions of the sort listed in the section of this book called 'What Most Doctors Don't Ask'.

For even within a very time-limited consultation it is possible to gather at least some information on the life context of a patient's symptoms by opening a consultation with a friendly general question such as 'How are things going?' – giving time for the patient to offer more than just a superficial answer.

When a patient reports symptoms, ask 'Had anything been troubling you before the symptoms started?'

Allow yourself to reflect on and share with the patient any possible symbolic or metaphorical dimension to a patient's symptoms, relating to their current life problems and circumstances.

Example: itching or sensitive skin:

"Anything you've been itching to do?" "Anything you've been feeling particularly sensitive to recently?"

Example: stomach, digestive or bowel symptoms:

"Anything you've found hard to stomach/digest/get out of your system recently?"

Ask for and make notes of *dates* – not just the patient's date of birth but the birth and/or death dates of relatives, siblings or spouses. You can do this in the course of asking about diseases in the family such as diabetes, cancer or heart disease.

Be aware of the *timing* of appointments made by patients – these may coincide with the timing of significant events such as births and deaths of people whom the patient identifies or feels a strong connection with.

Be aware that *genetic* explanations of illness may *disguise something completely different* – a strong psychological feeling towards and/or identification with a member of the patient's family. The fact that illnesses are transmitted across generations does not mean that the mode of transmission is principally genetic.

Always find a way to ask the patient what's been going on in their mind in relation to their symptoms, for example the question:

"What sort of thoughts and feelings tend to accompany your symptoms and what thoughts do you tend to have about them?"

Menstruation, Migraine and Meaning - A Short Lesson in 'Life Doctoring'

The following case offers a further example for biomedical doctors, emphasising the importance of (1) asking the patient *different type of questions* to those they might normally ask a patient (2) being alert to *symbolic* dimensions of a patient's symptoms and (3) seeing symbolic dimensions also to their own medical knowledge of a particular condition and its physiology (both in its typical and atypical manifestations in a given patient).

The aim is to show how taking this Life Medical approach can prove far more effective than simply approaching this condition in a standard way, e.g. by prescribing medications without consideration of *either* the life-context in which a patient's symptoms or condition emerged, its life meaning for the patient and the individual significance of both its typical and/or atypical aspects.

Case Example 7

The patient: a married woman in her late thirties who suffered from migraine for almost twenty years, at first irregular and non-menstrual related and then later becoming regular and menstrually related.

Questions to the patient:

When did the symptoms first occur?

The patient experienced her first, non-menstrual migraine during a stay at home from university during the summer holidays.

What were the most important life encounters, events, experiences or dilemmas preceding the onset of symptoms?

In this period she was effectively given the responsibility of 'head' of the family by her parents – having to both sort out family affairs and also take care of an elderly relative who she found quite repugnant.

Was there any sort of underlying mood accompanying the symptoms?

Yes, one of general negativity toward the tasks with which she was burdened but also guilt about her own negative feelings.

What did the symptoms force the patient to do, stop her doing or allow her to do?

The first strong migraine made it impossible for the patient to perform the tasks relegated to her by her parents. They forced her to spend days in a darkened room. In this way they also allowed her to take 'time out' from her tasks and give time to herself.

At what times do the symptoms tend to recur, intensify or diminish?

The patient's migraines had continued to recur irregularly for some years after the initial episode. Sometime after she embarked on her chosen career as a university lecturer, she got together with the partner she later married. The couple decided against having children because neither felt a need or wish to have a family. It was around this time that her migraines first began to recur regularly each month, before the onset of menstruation.

What did the patient do in response to her symptoms?

Taking medications in order to alleviate her symptoms sufficiently to able to 'function' in her work most of the time.

How did the symptoms, and the thoughts and feelings around them, affect the patient's life, work and relationships?

At first the patient's main aim was to use medication in order to not to let her migraines affect her work, which was an important medium of self-actualisation for her. As for her relationship however, though her husband had shared her choice to not have children, with the help of her psychotherapist the patient realised that she harboured some resentment about his seeming emotional indifference to the decision. After being encouraged by the therapist to feel her own feelings about her decision more deeply in her body – and to discuss the decision not to have children once again with her husband – the issue 'came to a head'. The patient was surprised to find that both she and her husband harboured feelings of sadness and loss at not having a family and that he was prepared to rethink should she change her mind. This removed her resentment toward what she had thought of as her husband's indifference and brought her closer together with him – whilst at the same time leaving her free to re-affirm her decision to stay childless. In the context of her long-term relationship, this did now *constitute* a concrete life decision in the true sense i.e. a definite choice between two available options.

What beliefs does the patient hold about their symptoms and the right way to respond to them?

The patient initially appeared to accept the standard socio-cultural beliefs made use of in the advertising propaganda put out by the pharmaceutical industry – beliefs which many doctors themselves are complicit in following. A principle belief is that with the help of the right 'off the counter' or prescription pill, patch, tampon, cream or pharmaceutical concoction there is never a need to not go sprightly and cheerfully out of the house and into the world and to stay economically active – whether you suffer from backaches, joint pains, headaches or even cyclical pre-menstrual symptoms. Indeed this applies particularly to menstruating women, who are given a graphic message through advertising that there is no need to not feel full of energy and unencumbered by the monthly 'curse'. Yet for a woman who is aware of her bodily and emotional needs, menstruation is a time to feel her body more fully and in this way also 'come back to herself', listen inwardly to her body and either grieve or rejoice that no child is on the way.

The menstrual cycle of course, follows the lunar cycle i.e. a healthy and natural cycle that all living beings are influenced by: a cycle of waxing and waning. This is one of many natural cycles – the cycle of expansion and contracting that can even be observed in the amoeba, the natural cycle of waking and sleeping, and a no less natural cycle of moving out into the world on the one hand, and withdrawing into one's self and body on the other.

Without phases of contraction no child would be born naturally. And without 'coming back to' or 'going down into' ourselves and our bodies we cannot feel ourselves or our bodies fully – and thus go out into the world and relate to others out of a fully re-embodied and authentic sense of self.

Current Westernised societies with their 24/7 culture however, no longer adhere to these cycles or natural rhythms and instead impose a constant 'forward' and 'out-going' movement as a normative way of living – negating the value of introspection, contraction or withdrawal from the world as unwelcome or even unhealthy and pathological conditions. That is why it is not surprising that both minor ailments such as headaches, colds and flues or even highly painful or discomforting symptoms or illnesses are so often needed as a 'cure' for what is effectively a *pathological* cultural norm – being the only socially acceptable way for individuals to break free of it – even if only by forcing individuals to take time out in which there is nothing to do but feel their bodies and thereby their own selves more fully – to *give time* to them.

Is there any positive and healthy side to the different mood and sense of self accompanying a patient's bodily symptoms – or to what their symptoms force or allow them permission to do – or not to do?

Are there any other ways in which the patient could give expression in their life to this positive and healthy side of their symptoms – without needing those symptoms as a spur to do so?

With the help of her psychotherapist – acting in the role of 'Life Doctor' – the patient herself quickly realised that she had deprived herself all her life of the benefits of a natural and healthy cycle of expansion and contraction. This was a breakthrough for the patient. It allowed her to recognise that the migraines – particularly when *not* medicated – forced her to slow down, to spend time with herself without working, reading, talking or distracting herself in other ways. She wondered whether this was what her body was trying to cure her of through her 'illness' and decided to see what happened if she started using this cure independently of the illness itself – for example by pacing herself more, allowing herself more time to not 'do' and just be, taking breaks instead of hurrying from one task to the other etc. So even though she continued to work very hard she no longer allowed the needs of work to dictate the natural rhythm of her day – and of her body – but began following her own. Even when she had to work 14-hour days she still made time to intersperse tasks with short breaks during which she allowed herself to be more consciously aware of her body and how she was feeling. About 3 weeks after changing her daily habits in this way – and doing so without feeling *guilty* for no longer following culturally imposed norms – she experienced her first migraine-free onset of menstruation in 15 years. Through her illness and the insights that also 'came to a head' through it, she hasn't had a migraine since – not because it was medically 'cured' but because she allowed the illness itself to help her 'cure' and overcome *unhealthy beliefs and an unhealthy way of living.*

What symbolic dimensions can be seen in the patient's symptoms and their history and what light do they shed on both menstrually and non-menstrually related migraine?

Both the symptoms of menstruation and those of migraine ask people to take 'time out' from their regular routines – or rather to take 'time in' – time to go into themselves, just be with and feel themselves more fully from within. The typical symptoms of migraine – painful headache, nausea, feeling sick and vomiting, sensitivity to light and noise can be seen as having two principal symbolic dimensions. One is the service they perform in bringing the effects of a culturally normative but essentially unnatural and unhealthy way of living 'to a head' – through painful headaches. The other symbolic dimension has to do with how sufferers respond to migraine attacks, which is often by shutting themselves off in a darkened room – as if recreating a *womb* for themselves shielded from light and sound.

Herein lies a symbolic clue, not only to the frequency of so-called 'menstrual migraine' in women, but also to the unmet needs of male sufferers. In the specific context of the patient referred to, it is symbolically interesting to note also that hers was a profession – university lecturer – focussed on use of the head. And in an age in which sedentary 'service' professions and mental work dominates over farming or different forms of manual work, there is a far greater tendency for individuals to lose touch with their bodies – and in particular with the so-called 'gut brain' as opposed to the 'head brain'. For this, like the uterus, is located in the abdomen – which contains more nerve cells than the brain. Finally it is to be noted again that the patient's first episode of migraine, albeit non-menstrual, occurred at a time when, though supposedly on holiday, her time was filled with tasks that effectively demanded that she take on the role of *parent* in relation to her own parents. In this context, her migraine can be seen as serving an important and healthy balancing role by making her withdraw to a darkened room – thus allowing and encouraging her to both avoid and recover from the parental tasks placed on her by placing herself back in the position of a baby in a protective womb.

Though it is a not an uncommon condition, medical literature and practice never attempt to see any symbolic connection between 'menstrual' or 'menstrually related' migraine on the one hand, and a women's relation to both her periods and to having or not having children. This is of no small significance in a time and a culture where women are under greater pressure than ever either to manage the highly demanding and stressful role of 'working mother' or else to put the interests of their careers and employers ahead of motherhood. Of symbolic note here is also the fact that the use of standard hormonal contraceptives to avoid pregnancy are known to worsen the symptoms of menstrual migraine and are specifically contra-indicated for women over thirty five i.e. precisely those women reaching a critical life phase in terms of deciding whether to stay childless or not.

PART 6
APPENDICES

1. Death by Doctoring

"In the United States – where 40,000 people are shot to death each year – the chance of getting "killed" by a doctor is three times greater than being killed by a gun." Ben Ong

"An article written by Dr Barbara Starfield, MD, MPH, of the John Hopkins School of Hygiene and Public Health, shows that medical errors may be the third leading cause of death in the United States. The report apparently shows there are 2,000 deaths/year from unnecessary surgery; 7000 deaths/year from medication errors in hospitals; 20,000 deaths/year from other errors in hospitals; 80,000 deaths/year from infections in hospitals; 106,000 deaths/year from non-error, adverse effects of medications – these total up to 225,000 deaths per year in the US from iatrogenic causes which ranks these deaths as the third killer. Iatrogenic is a term used when a patient dies as a direct result of treatments by a physician, whether it is from misdiagnosis of the ailment or from adverse drug reactions used to treat the illness (drug reactions are the most common cause). Based on the findings of one major study, medical errors kill some 44,000 people in U.S. hospitals each year. Another study puts the number much higher, at 98,000. Even using the lower estimate, more people die from medical mistakes each year than from highway accidents, breast cancer, or AIDS. *And deaths from medication errors that take place both in and out of hospitals are said to be more than 7,000 annually."* www.cancure.org/medical_errors.htm

Indeed the statistics point to medicine actually being the *first and leading cause of death.* For in the 2001 annual death rate from heart disease in the U.S. was 699,697; and the cancer death rate was 553,251.

Compare this with the following table for 'iatrogenic' or medically induced deaths:

Adverse Drug Reactions	106,000
Medical error	98,000
Bedsores	115,000
Infection	88,000
Malnutrition	108,800
Outpatients	199,000
Unnecessary Procedures	37,136
Total	**783,936**

Projected over a ten-year period this gives us a figure of almost 7.84 million – more than all the deaths from all the wars fought by America. Note also the projected ten-year statistics for 'unnecessary events' i.e. unnecessary medical intervention, along with the corresponding figures for adverse results stemming from these unnecessary treatment 'procedures'.

Unnecessary Events

Hospitalization	89 million	17 million
Procedures	75 million	15 million
TOTAL	164 million	

As Ben Ong notes, this table indicates that *56% of the population of the United States, have been treated unnecessarily by the medical industry* - in other words, nearly 50,000 people per day.

ben.ong@cure-prostate.com

"The National Academies website published an article titled "Preventing Death and Injury From Medical Errors Requires Dramatic, System-Wide Changes." which you can read online at 'www4.nationalacademies.org/news.nsf/isbn/0309068371?Ope nDocument' or the book "To Err Is Human: Building a Safer Health System" at www.nap.edu/books/0309068371/html/ - These show medical errors as a leading cause of death. Based on the findings of one major study, medical errors kill some 44,000 people in U.S. hospitals each year. Another study puts the number much higher, at 98,000. Even using the lower estimate, more people die from medical mistakes each year than from highway accidents, breast cancer, or AIDS. And deaths from medication errors that take place both in and out of hospitals are said to be more than 7,000 annually."

www.cancure.org/medical_errors.htm

Prescription Drugs – Leading Killer in USA

"... a statistical study of hospital deaths in the U.S. conducted at the University of Toronto revealed that pharmaceutical drugs kill more people every year than are killed in traffic accidents. The study is said to show that more than two million American hospitalized patients suffered a serious adverse drug reaction (ADR) within the 12-month period of the study and, of these, over 100,000 died as a result. The researchers found that over 75 per cent of these ADRs were dose-dependent, which suggests they were due to the inherent toxicity of the drugs rather than to allergic reactions.

The data did not include fatal reactions caused by accidental overdoses or errors in administration of the drugs. If these had been included, it is estimated that another 100,000 deaths would be added to the total every year. The researchers concluded that ADRs are now the fourth leading cause of death in the United States after heart disease, cancer, and stroke."

www.cancure.org/medical_errors.htm

"Getting the wrong drug or the wrong dosage kills hundreds or thousands of people each year, with many times that number getting injured ... Even higher than the number of people who die from medication errors is the number of people who die from medication, period. Even when a prescription drug is dispensed properly, there's no guarantee it won't end up killing you. A remarkable study in the Journal of the American Medical Association revealed that prescription drugs kill around 106,000 people in the US every year, which ranks prescription drugs as

the fourth leading cause of death. Furthermore, each year sees 2,216,000 serious adverse drug reactions (defined as "those that required hospitalization, were permanently disabling, or resulted in death"). The authors of this 1998 study performed a meta-analysis on 39 previous studies covering 32 years. They factored out such things as medication errors, abuse of prescription drugs, and adverse reactions not considered serious. Plus, the study involved only people who had either been hospitalized due to drug reactions or who experienced reactions while in the hospital. People who died immediately (and, thus, never went to the hospital) and those whose deaths weren't realized to be due to prescription drugs were not included, so the true figure is probably higher. Four years later, another study in the JAMA warned:

Patient exposure to new drugs with unknown toxic effects may be extensive. Nearly 20 million patients in the United States took at least 1 of the 5 drugs withdrawn from the market between September 1997 and September 1998. Three of these 5 drugs were new, having been on the market for less than 2 years. Seven drugs approved since 1993 and subsequently withdrawn from the market have been reported as possibly contributing to 1002 deaths.

Examining warnings added to drug labels through the years, the study's authors found that of the new chemical entities approved from 1975 to 1999, 10 percent "acquired a new black box warning or were withdrawn from the market" by 2000. Using some kind of high-falutin' statistical process, they estimate that the "probability of a new drug acquiring black box warnings or being withdrawn from the market over 25 years was 20%." A statement released by one of the study's co-authors, Sidney Wolfe, MD, Director of Public Citizen's Health Studies Group, warned:

'In 1997, 39 new drugs were approved by the FDA. As of now [May 2002], five of them (Rezulin, Posicor, Duract, Raxar and Baycol) have been taken off the market and an additional two (Trovan, an antibiotic and Orgaran, an anticoagulant) have had new box warnings. Thus, seven drugs approved that year (18% of the 39 drugs approved) have already been withdrawn or had a black box warning in just four years after approval. Based on our study, 20% of drugs will be withdrawn or have a black box warning within 25 years of coming on the market. The drugs approved in 1997 have already almost "achieved" this in only four years — with 21 years to go.' How does this happen? Before the FDA approves a new drug, it must undergo clinical trials. These trials aren't performed by the FDA, though — they're done by the drug companies themselves. These trials often use relatively few patients, and they usually select patients most likely to react well to the drug. On top of that, the trials are often for a short period of time (weeks), even though real-world users may be on a drug for months or years at a time. Dr. Wolfe points out that even when adverse effects show up during clinical trials, the drugs are sometimes released anyway, and they end up being taken off the market because of those same adverse effects. Postmarketing reporting of adverse effects isn't much better. The FDA runs a program to collect reports of problems with drugs, but compliance is voluntary. The generally accepted estimate in the medical community is that a scant 10 percent of individual instances of adverse effects are reported to the FDA, which

would mean that the problem is ten times worse than we currently believe. Drugs aren't released when they've been proven safe; they're released when enough FDA bureaucrats — many of whom have worked for the pharmaceutical companies or will work for them in the future — can be convinced that it's kinda safe. Basically, the use of prescription drugs by the general public can be seen as widespread, long-term clinical trials to determine their true safety. We are all guinea pigs."

From *50 Things You're Not Supposed to Know* by Russ Kick, published by The Disinformation Company Ltd. http://www.disinfo.com/

Note: *Heroin* - that most notorious of 'illegal', 'non-prescription' drugs, was originally developed by the pharmaceutical company BAYER for use as a legal prescription drug.

"The majority of the cancer patients in this country die because of chemotherapy, which does not cure breast, colon or lung cancer. This has been documented for over a decade and nevertheless doctors still utilize chemotherapy to fight these tumors." Allen Levin, MD, UCSF

"Several full-time scientists at the McGill Cancer Center sent to 118 doctors, all experts on lung cancer, a questionnaire to determine the level of trust they had in the therapies they were applying; they were asked to imagine that they themselves had contracted the disease and which of the six current experimental therapies they would choose. 79 doctors answered, 64 of them

said that they would not consent to undergo any treatment containing cis-platinum – one of the common chemotherapy drugs they used – while 58 out of 79 believed that all the experimental therapies above were not accepted because of the ineffectiveness and the elevated level of toxicity of chemotherapy."

Philip Day, *Cancer: why we're still dying to know the truth*, Credence 2000

"If I were to contract cancer, I would never turn to a certain standard for the therapy of this disease. Cancer patients who stay away from these centers have some chance to make it."

Professor Gorge Mathe, *Scientific Medicine Stymied*, Medicines Nouvelles, Paris, 1989

"Dr. Hardin Jones, lecturer at the University of California, after having analyzed for many decades statistics on cancer survival, has come to this conclusion: '... when not treated, the patients do not get worse or they even get better'. The unsettling conclusions of Dr. Jones have never been refuted".

Walter Last, "The Ecologist", Vol. 28, no. 2, March-April 1998

ADVERSE DRUG REACTIONS: How Serious Is the Problem and How Often and Why Does It Occur?

"Although some adverse drug reactions are not very serious, others cause the death, hospitalization, or serious injury of more than 2 million people in the United states each year, including more than 100,000 fatalities. In fact, adverse drug reactions are one of the leading causes of death in the United States.' Most of

the time, these dangerous events could and should have been avoided. Even the less drastic reactions, such as change in mood, loss of appetite, and nausea, may seriously diminish the quality of life.

Despite the fact that more adverse reactions occur in patients 60 or older, the odds of suffering an adverse drug reaction really begin to increase even before age 50. Almost half (49.5%) of Food and Drug Administration (FDA) reports of deaths from adverse drug reactions and 61% of hospitalizations from adverse drug reactions were in people younger than 60.2 Many physical changes that affect the way the body can handle drugs actually begin in people in their thirties, but the increased prescribing of drugs does not begin for most people until they enter their fifties. By then, the amount of prescription drug use starts increasing significantly, and therefore the odds of having an adverse drug reaction also increase. The risk of an adverse drug reaction is about 33% higher in people aged 50 to 59 than it is in people aged 40."

Adverse Reactions to Drugs Cause Hospitalization of 1.5 Million Americans Each Year:

"An analysis of numerous studies in which the cause of hospitalization was determined found that approximately 1.5 million hospitalizations a year were caused by adverse drug reactions. This means that every day more than 9,000 patients have adverse drug reactions so serious that they need to be admitted to American hospitals. Although the rate of drug-induced hospitalization is higher in older adults (an average of

about 10% of all hospitalizations for older adults are caused by adverse drug reactions) because they use more drugs, a significant proportion of hospitalizations for children is also caused by adverse drug reactions. In a review of more than 6,500 admissions of children to five different hospitals, 2.0% were prompted by adverse drug reactions."

Adverse Reactions Occur to 770,000 People a Year During Hospitalization

"In addition to the 1.5 million people a year who are admitted to the hospital because of adverse drug reactions, an additional three quarters of a million people a year develop an adverse reaction after they are hospitalized. According to national projection, based on a study involving adverse drug reactions developing in almost 800,000 patients a year, more than 2,000 patients a day, suffer an adverse event caused by drugs once they are admitted. Many of the reactions in the patients studied were serious, even life-threatening, and included cardiac arrhythmias, kidney failure, bleeding, and dangerously low blood pressure. People with these adverse reactions had an almost twofold higher risk of death compared to otherwise comparable hospitalized patients who did not have a drug reaction. Most importantly, according to the researchers, almost 50% of these adverse reactions were preventable. Among the kinds of preventable problems were adverse interactions between drugs that should not have been prescribed together (hundreds of these are listed in Chapter 3 of this book), known allergies to drugs that had not been asked about before the patients got a

prescription, and excessively high doses of drugs prescribed without considering the patient's weight and kidney functions.

Thus, adding the number of people with adverse drug reactions so serious that they require hospitalization to those in which the adverse reaction was "caused" by the hospitalization, more than 2.2 million people a year, or 6,000 patients a day, suffer these adverse reactions. In both situations, many of these drug-induced problems should have been prevented."

Dr. Tim O'Shea, www.cancer-healing.com/pharma_pills.php

"...at least 250,000 people have attempted suicide worldwide because of Prozac alone and that at least 25,000 have succeeded."

Professor David Healy

2. Extracts from
'The Way Toward Health' by Jane Roberts

If people become ill, it is quite fashionable to say that the immunity system has temporarily failed – yet the body itself knows that certain 'dis-eases' are healthy reactions. The body does not recognise <u>diseases as diseases</u> in usually understood terms. It regards all activity as experience, as a momentary condition of life, as a balancing situation.

It is ... fashionable to say that men and women have conscious minds, subconscious minds and unconscious minds – but there is no such thing as an unconscious mind. The body consciousness is <u>highly conscious</u>. You are simply not conscious of it.

You might say [instead] that varying portions of your own consciousness operate at different speeds. Translations between one portion of consciousness and another go on constantly, so that information is translated from one 'speed' to another.

....

Many psychiatrists and psychologists now realise that a disturbed client cannot be helped sufficiently unless the individual is considered along with his or her relationship to the family unit.

The same idea applies to physical illness as well. It is possible, however, to carry this idea even further, so that a person in poor health <u>should be</u> seen by the physician in relationship to the family and also in relationship to the environment. Old-time family doctors understood the patient's sensitivity to family members and to the environment, of course, and they often felt a lively sympathy and understanding that the practitioners of modern medicine often seem to have forgotten.

....

Modern medical science largely considers the human body to be a kind of mechanical model, a sort of vehicle like a car that needs to be checked by a garage every so often.

As an automobile is put together at an assembly line, so the body is seen as a very efficient machine put together in nature's 'factory'. If all the parts are in their proper place, and functioning smoothly, then the machine should give as excellent a service as any well-running automobile – or so it seems.

All of the automobile's parts, however, are alone responsible for its operations so long as it has a responsible driver. There are, however, hidden relationships that exist between various parts of the body – and the parts themselves are hardly mechanical. They change in every moment.

The heart is often described as a type of pump. With the latest developments in modern technology, there are all kinds of heart operations that can be performed, even the use of heart transplants. In many cases, even when hearts are repaired through medical technology, the same trouble reoccurs at a later date, or the patient recovers only to fall prey to a different, nearly fatal or fatal disease. This is not always the case by any means, but when such a person does recover fully, and maintains good health, it is because [their] beliefs, attitudes and feelings have changed for the better, and because the person 'has a heart' again; in other words because the patient himself has regained the will to live.

Many people who have heart trouble feel that they have 'lost the heart' for life. They may feel broken-hearted for many reasons. They may feel heartless, or imagine themselves to be so cold-hearted that they punish themselves literally by trying to lose their heart.

With many people having such difficulties, the addition of love in the environment may work far better than any heart operation. A new pet given to a bereaved individual has saved more people from needing heart operations than any physician. In other words, a 'love transplant' in the environment may work far better overall than a heart-transplant operation, or a bypass, or whatever; in such ways the heart is allowed to heal itself.

People have been taught to trust 275a picture of what is happening in their bodies, and cautioned not to trust their own feelings. Some public-service announcements stress the 'fact' that the individual can be gravely threatened by high blood pressure, for example, even though he or she feels in excellent health.

In many cases people exercise quite simply because they are afraid of what will happen if they do not. They may run to avoid heart disease, for example, whilst their own fear can <u>help</u> to promote the very eventuality they fear.

The body's health is an expression of inner well-being. Poor health is an expression also, and it may serve many purposes. It goes without saying that some people become ill rather than change their activities and their environments. They may also become ill, of course, to <u>force</u> themselves to make such changes.

I do not mean to imply that exercise is detrimental to good health. It is true, however, that the reason you exercise is more important than the exercises that you do perform. The reason can promote your good health or actually impede it.

....

The concept of survival of the fittest has had a considerable detrimental effect in many areas of human activity – particularly the realm of medical ideology and practice.

Politically as well as medically, such distortions have led to unfortunate conditions; the Aryan supremacy biological ideas fostered in the second world war, the concentration upon 'the perfect body', and other distortions. The idea of the ideal body has often been held up to the populace at large, and this often sets forth a stylised 'perfect' physique that actually could be matched by few individuals.

Any variations are frowned upon, and any birth defects considered in the most suspicious of lights. Some schools of thought then, have it that only the genetically superior should be allowed to reproduce, and there are scientists who believe that all defects can be eliminated through judicious genetic planning.

The handicapped are often given messages, even by the medical profession, that make them feel like misfits, unworthy to survive.

....

Your ideas about yourself are, again vital in the larger context of a healthy lifetime. The condition of your heart is affected, for example, by your own feelings about it. If you consider yourself to be cold-hearted or heartless, those feelings will have a significant effect upon that physical organ. If you feel broken-hearted then you will also have that feeling reflected in one way or another in the physical organ itself.

.... each individual also has many options open. Everyone who feels broken-hearted does not necessarily die of heart failure for example. The subject of health cannot be considered in an isolated fashion ... each person will try to fulfil their own unique abilities, and to 'fill out' the experience of life as fully as possible.

If an individual is hampered in that attempt strongly and persistently, then the dissatisfaction and frustration will be transformed into a lack of physical exuberance and vitality. There is always an unending reservoir of energy at the command of each person however, regardless of circumstances. ...

....

Thoughts and beliefs do indeed bring about physical alterations. They can even – and often do – change genetic messages.

There are diseases that people believe are inherited, carried from one generation to another by a faulty genetic communication. Obviously, many people with, for example, a genetic heritage of arthritis, do not come down with the disease themselves, while others indeed are so afflicted. The difference is one of belief.

The people who have accepted the suggestion uncritically that they will inherit such a malady do then seem to inherit it: they experience the symptoms. Actually the belief itself may have turned a healthy genetic message into an unhealthy one.

....

...pain and suffering are also obviously vital, living sensations – and therefore are a part of the body's repertoire of possible feelings and sensual experience. They are also a sign, therefore, of life's vitality, and are in themselves often responsible for a return to health when they act as learning communications.

Many diseases are often health-promoting processes. Chicken pox, measles and other like diseases in childhood in their own way 'naturally inoculate' the body, so that it is able to handle other elements that are a part of the body and the body's environment.

When civilised children are medically inoculated against such diseases ... to an important extent the natural protective processes are impeded. Such children may not come down with the disease against which they are medically protected, then – but they may indeed therefore become 'prey' to other diseases later in life that would not otherwise have occurred.

I am not advising people to refuse to have their children vaccinated, since you now have to take vaccination into consideration because of its prominence in society. It is very possible however, that science itself will in time discover the unfortunate side effects of many such procedures, and begin to reevaluate the entire subject.

....

... no person dies ahead of his or her time. The individual chooses the time of death. It is true however, that many cancers and conditions such as AIDS result because the immunity system has been so tampered with that the body has not been allowed to follow through with its own balancing act.

Again, however, no individual dies of cancer or AIDS, or any other condition, until they themselves have set the time.

...no consciousness considers death an <u>end or a disaster</u>, but views it instead as a means to the continuation of ... existence.

....

People with life-threatening diseases ... often feel that further growth, development, or expansion are highly difficult, if not impossible to achieve at a certain point in their lives. Often there are complicated family relationships that the person does not know how to handle ... In all cases, however, the need for value fulfilment, expression, and creativity are so important to life that when these are threatened, life itself is at least momentarily weakened. Innately, each person does realise that there is life after death, and in some instances such people realise that it is indeed time to move to another level of reality, to die and set out again with another brand new world.

Often, seriously ill people quite clearly recognise such feelings but they have been taught not to speak of them. The desire to die is considered cowardly, even evil, by some religions – and yet behind that desire lies all of the vitality of the will to life, which may already be seeking new avenues of expression and meaning.

There are those who come down with one serious disease – say heart trouble – who are cured through a heart transplant or other medical procedure, only to fall prey to another, seemingly unrelated disease, such as cancer. It would relieve the minds of family and friends, however if they understood that the individual involved did not 'fall prey' to the disease, and that he or she was not a victim in usual terms.

This does not mean that anyone consciously decides to get such-and-such a disease, but it does mean that some people instinctively realise that their own development does now demand another new framework of existence.

Much loneliness results when people who know they are going to die feel unable to communicate with loved ones for fear of hurting their feelings. Still other kinds of individuals will live long productive lives even while their physical mobility or health is most severely impaired. They will still feel that they had work to do, or that they were needed ...

....

Many cancer patients have martyr-like characteristics, often putting up with undesirable situations or conditions for years.

They feel powerless, unable to change, yet unwilling to stay in the same position. The most important point is to arouse such a person's belief in his or her strength and power. In many instances these people shrug their shoulders, saying "What will happen, will happen," but they do not physically struggle against their situation.

It is also vital that these patients are not overly medicated, for oftentimes the side effects of some cancer-eradicating drugs are dangerous in themselves. There has been some success with people who imagine that the cancer is instead some hated enemy or monster or foe, which is then banished with mental mock battles over a period of time. While the technique does have its advantages, it also pits one portion of the self against the other. It is much better to imagine say, the cancer cells being neutralised by some imaginary wand.

Doctors might suggest that a patient relax and then ask himself or herself what kind of inner fantasy would best serve the healing process. Instant images may come to mind at once, but if success is not achieved immediately, have the patient try again, for in almost all cases <u>some</u> inner picture will be perceived.

Behind the entire problem, however, is the fear of using one's full power or energy. Cancer patients most usually feel an inner impatience as they sense their own need for future expansion and development, only to feel it thwarted.

Again, we cannot generalise overmuch, but many persons know quite well that they are not sure whether they want to live or die. The overabundance of cancer cells represents nevertheless the need for expression and expansion – the only arena left open – or so it would seem.

Such a person must also contend with society's unfortunate ideas about the disease in general, so that many cancer patients end up isolated or alone. As in almost all cases of disease however, if it were possible to have a kind of 'thought transplant' operation, the disease would quickly vanish.

Consciously you might want to express certain abilities, whilst unconsciously you are afraid of doing so.

....

For all of life's seeming misfortunes, development, fulfilment and accomplishment far outweigh death, diseases and disasters. Starting over can be done – by anyone in any situation, and it will bring about some beneficial effects regardless of previous conditions.

Behind all maladies, in the most basic manner lies the need for expression, and when people feel that their areas of growth are being curtailed, then they instigate actions meant to clear the road, so to speak.

Before health problems show up there is almost always a loss of self-respect or expression.

In the matter of the disease called AIDS, for example, you have groups of homosexuals, many 'coming out of the closet' for the first time, taking part in organisations that promote their cause, and suddenly faced by the suspicions and distrust of many other portions of the population.

The struggle to express themselves, and their own unique abilities and characteristics, drives them on, and yet is all too frequently thwarted by the ignorance and misunderstanding that surrounds them. You end up with something like a <u>psychological contagion</u>. The people involved begin to feel even more depressed as they struggle to combat the prejudice against them. Many of them almost hate themselves. For all their seeming bravado, they fear that they are indeed unnatural members of the species.

These beliefs break down the immunity system and bring about the symptoms so connected with the disease. AIDS is a social phenomenon to that extent, expressing the deep dissatisfactions, doubts and angers of a prejudiced-against segment of society.

Whatever physical changes occur, happen because the will to live is weakened. AIDS is a kind of biological protest, as if the homosexuals are saying: "You may as well kill us. We might be better off than the way you treat us now" ...

The attitude of doctors and nurses towards the handling of such patients shows only too clearly not only their fear of the disease itself, but their fear of homosexuality, which has been considered evil and forbidden by many religions.

Yet AIDS can be acquired by those who are not homosexuals, but who have similar problems. It is a great error to segregate some individuals, like a modern colony of lepers.

Many other conditions that seem to be spread by viruses or contagions are also related to the problems of society in the same manner, and when these conditions are righted the diseases themselves largely vanish. It should be remembered that it is the beliefs and feelings of the patients that largely determine the effectiveness of any medical procedures, techniques or medications.

Unfortunately, the entire picture surrounding health and disease is a largely negative one, in which even preventative medicine can have severe drawbacks, since it often recommends drugs or techniques to attack a problem not only before the problem emerges, but simply in case it emerges.

Many of the public-health announcements routinely publicise the specific symptoms of various diseases, almost as if laying out maps of diseases for medical consumers to follow.

The body's own healing processes are forever active however – which is why I so strongly advise them being relied upon along with whatever medical help seems appropriate. But the individual, even as a patient, must always have a choice, and the right to refuse any treatment being offered.

....

You cannot divorce philosophy from life, for your thoughts and opinions give your life its meaning and impetus. There are some people who believe that life is meaningless, that it has no purpose, and that its multitudinous parts fell together through the workings of chance alone. Obviously I am speaking of scientific dogma, but such dogma is far more religious than scientific, for it also expects to be believed without proof, on faith alone.

All of life is seen as heading for extinction in any case. The entire concept of a soul, life after death, or even life from one generation to the next, becomes doubtful, to say the least. In such a philosophical world it would seem that man has no power at all.

... those concepts can have a hand in the development of would-be suicides, particularly of a young age, for they seem to effectively block a future.

....

For centuries it was taken for granted that God was on the side of the strongest, richest nation. Surely, it seemed, if a country was poor or downtrodden, it was because God made it so.

Such ideas literally held people in chains, fostering slavery and other inhumane practices. The same unfortunately applies to Eastern concepts of nirvana and to the Christian idea of heaven.

There are many differences between the ideas of nirvana and heaven, but each has been used, not only to justify suffering, but also to teach people to seek pain.

Quite ordinary people often believe, then, that suffering itself is a way towards personal development and spiritual knowledge. In matters of health, such beliefs can have most unfortunate results. They are often responsible for needless sacrifices of physical organs in imprudent operations.

Some individuals become anxious and worried if they think they are too happy – for them it means they are not paying sufficiently for their sins. They may be threatened by some undeniable danger, until finally, in one way or another they seek out their own punishment once again – wondering all the time why they are so frequently besieged by poor health or disease.

This kind of syndrome can affect individuals, families, and to some extent entire nations. They mitigate directly against man's health, survival and exuberance.

Constant fears about … catastrophes can also fall under this classification.

This is true of individuals, but it also applies to many so-called survival groups, who congregate in one or another portion of the country.

Most such people expect a period of chaotic time, in which all laws are broken down. Another version stresses the economic area, foreseeing the collapse of the economy, anarchy, and other conditions that pit one individual against another. Some use religious dogma and others rely upon scientific dogma to prove their cases ...

Good mental or physical health can hardly flourish in such conditions.

Such ideas affect every level of life, from the most microscopic onward. It is not that plants understand your ideas in usual terms, but that they do indeed pick up your intent, and in the area of world survival, they have a stake.

I do not want to romanticise nonhuman life either, or to overestimate its resources, but nature also has its own ways – and in those ways it constantly works towards the survival of life in general. Nature may not bail you out, but it will always be there, adding its own vitality and strength to the overall good and health of the planet.

Communication flashes between viruses and microbes, and they can change in the wink of an eye. Once again then, ideas of the most optimistic nature are the biologically pertinent ones.

....

This is a good place to bring up some extreme food practices, such as over-fasting and an obsession with so-called natural foods. I am not talking about a natural and healthy interest in the purity of foodstuffs, but of a worrisome overconcern.

Behind many such attitudes is the idea that the body itself is unworthy, and that starving it somehow cuts down on the appetites of the flesh. You usually end up with a flurry of different types of diets.

Some concentrate almost exclusively on protein, some on carbohydrates – particularly rice – but in any case the large natural range of foods and nutrients are cut out.

This keeps the body in a state of constant turmoil. Some people are so convinced, in fact, that eating is wrong that they diet until they become ravenously hungry, then overeat and force themselves to vomit up the residue.

Other people, in a well-meaning attempt to watch their weight, skip their breakfasts entirely – a very poor procedure.

It is far better to eat moderate amounts of food in all of the food ranges, and to consume smaller portions more often ... four light meals a day will overall serve you very well.

These food ideas are important, since they are often passed on from parents to children, and parents often use food as a way of rewarding a child's good behaviour, thus starting the youngster out towards the condition of overweight.

....

If you do have health problems, it is much better to look for their reason in your immediate experience ...

... try to understand that the particular dilemma of illness is not an event forced upon you by some other agency. Rather realise that to some extent or another your dilemma or your illness has been chosen by you ...

If you realise that your beliefs form your experience, then you do have a very good chance of changing your beliefs, and hence your experience.

You can discover what your own reasons are for choosing the dilemma or illness by being very honest with yourself. There is no need to feel guilty since you <u>meant very well</u> as you made each choice – only the choices were built upon beliefs that were beliefs and <u>not facts</u>.

If you are in serious difficulties of any kind, it may at first seem inconceivable, unbelievable or even scandalous to imagine that your problems are caused by your beliefs. In fact, the opposite may appear to be true. You might have lost a series of jobs, and it may seem quite clear to you that you are not to blame in any of these circumstances.

You may be in the middle of one or several unsatisfactory relationships, none of which seem to be caused by you, while instead you believe you are an unwilling victim or participant. You may have a dangerous drug or alcohol problem, or you may be married to someone who does.

In most cases, even the most severe illnesses or complicated living conditions are caused by an attempt to grow, develop or expand in the face of difficulties that appear to be insurmountable to one degree or another.

An individual will appear to be striving for some goal that appears blocked, and hence he or she uses all available energy and strength to circumnavigate the blockage.

[In fact] the blockage is usually a belief which needs to be understood or removed rather than bypassed.

....

You are not healthy ... no matter how robust your physical condition, if your relationships are unhealthy, unsatisfying, frustrating or hard to achieve. Whatever your situation is, it is a good idea to ask yourself <u>what you would do</u> if you were free of it. An alcoholic's wife might wish with all her heart that her husband would stop drinking – but if she suddenly asked herself what she would do, she might – surprisingly enough – feel a tinge of panic. On examination of her own thoughts and feelings, she might well discover that she was so frightened of not achieving her own goals that she actually encouraged her husband's alcoholism, so that she would not have to face her own 'failure'. Obviously this hypothetical situation is a quick example of what I mean, with no mention of the innumerable other beliefs and half-beliefs that would encircle the man's and the woman's relationship.

Each person is so unique that it is obviously impossible for me to discuss all of the innumerable strands of belief that form human experience .... you may discover not just one you, but several you's, so to speak, each pursuing certain purposes, and you may find out furthermore that some purposes cancel others out, whilst some are diametrically opposed to one another. Such cross-purposes, of course can lead to mental, spiritual, emotional and physical difficulties.

Large numbers of people do indeed live unsatisfactory lives, with many individuals seeking goals that are nearly unattainable because of the conglomeration of contradictory beliefs that vie for their attention. They are at cross-purposes with themselves.

Addendum: from 'The Individual and the Nature of Mass Events' – a Seth Book by Jane Roberts:

Many therefore "fall prey" to epidemics of one kind or another because they want to, though they might deny this quite vigorously.

I am speaking particularly of epidemics that are less than deadly, though danger is involved. In your times, hospitals, you must realize, are important parts of the community. They provide a social as well as a medical service. Many people are simply lonely, or overworked. Some are rebelling against commonly held ideas of competition. Flu epidemics become social excuses for much needed rest, therefore, and serve as face-saving devices so that the individual can hide from *themselves* their inner difficulties. In a way, such epidemics provide their own kind of fellowship – giving common meeting grounds for those of disparate circumstances. The [epidemics] serve as accepted states of illness, in which people are given an excuse for the rest or quiet self-examination they desperately need but do not feel entitled to otherwise.

I do not mean to assign any hint of accusation against those so involved, but mainly to state some of the reasons for such behavior. If you do not trust your nature, then any illness or disposition will be interpreted as an onslaught against health. Your body faithfully reflects your inner psychological reality. The nature of your emotions means that in the course of a lifetime you will experience the full range of feelings. Your subjective state has variety. Sometimes sad or depressing thoughts provide a refreshing change of pace, leading you to periods of quiet reflection, and to a quieting of the body so that it rests.

Fears, sometimes even seemingly irrational ones, can serve to rouse the body if you have been too lethargic, or have been in a rut psychologically or physically. If you trusted your nature you would be able to trust such feelings, and following their own rhythms and routes they would change into others. Ideally even illnesses are a part of the body's health, representing needed adjustments, and also following the needs of the subjective person at any given time.

3. Extracts from 'Medical Nemesis - The Expropriation of Health' by Ivan Illich

The medical establishment has become a major threat to health. The disabling impact of professional control over medicine has reached the proportions of an epidemic. *Iatrogenesis*, the name for this new epidemic, comes from *iatros*, the Greek word for 'physician', and *genesis*, meaning 'origin'.

A professional and physician-based health-care system that has grown beyond critical bounds is sickening for three reasons: it must produce clinical damage that outweighs its potential benefits; it cannot but enhance even as it obscures the political conditions that render society unhealthy; and it tends to expropriate the power of the individual to heal himself and shape his or her environment.

More and more people subconsciously know that they are sick and tired of their jobs and of their leisure passivities, but they want to hear the lie that physical illness relieves them of social and political responsibilities. They want their doctor to act as lawyer and priest. As a lawyer, the doctor exempts the patient from his normal duties and enables him to cash in on the insurance fund he was forced to build. As a priest, he becomes the patient's accomplice in creating the myth that he is an innocent victim of biological mechanisms rather than a lazy, greedy or envious deserter of a social struggle for control over the tools of production. Social life becomes a giving and receiving of therapy: medical, psychiatric, pedagogic or geriatric.

People who are angered, sickened and impaired by their industrial labour and leisure can escape only into a life under medical supervision and are thereby seduced or disqualified from political struggle for a healthier world.

Medicine has the authority to label one man's complaint a legitimate illness, to declare a second man sick though he does not himself complain, and to refuse a third social recognition of his pain, his disability and even his death. It is medicine which stamps some pain as 'merely subjective', some impairment as malingering, and some deaths – though not others – as suicide. The judge determines what is legal and who is guilty. The priest declares what is holy and who has broken a taboo. The physician decides what is a symptom and who is sick.

For rich and poor...life is reduced to a 'span', to a statistical phenomenon which, for better or worse, must be institutionally planned and shaped. This life-span is brought into existence with the pre-natal check-up...and it will end with a mark on a chart...

To be in good health means not only to be successful in coping with reality but also to enjoy the success; it means to be able to feel alive in pleasure and in pain; it means to cherish but also to risk survival. Health and suffering, as experienced sensations are phenomena that distinguish men from beasts. Only storybook lions are said to *suffer* and only pets to merit compassion when they are in ill-health.

Medicalisation constitutes a prolific bureaucratic programme based on the denial of each man's need to deal with pain, sickness and death. The modern medical enterprise represents an endeavour to do for people what their genetic and cultural heritage formerly equipped them to do for themselves. Medical civilization is planned and organized to kill pain, to eliminate sickness, and to abolish the need for an art of suffering and of dying.

Culture makes pain tolerable by interpreting its necessity; only pain perceived as curable is intolerable.

A myriad virtues express the different aspects of fortitude that traditionally enabled people to recognize painful sensations as a challenge and to shape their own experience accordingly. Patience, forbearance, courage, resignation, self-control, perseverance, and meekness each express a different colouring of the responses with which pain sensations were accepted, transformed into the experience of suffering and endured. Duty, love, fascination, routines, prayer, and compassion were some of the means that enabled pain to be borne with dignity.

The pupils of Hippocrates distinguished many kinds of disharmony, each of which caused its own type of pain...Pain might disappear in the process of healing, but this was certainly not the primary object of the...treatment. The Greeks did not even think about enjoying happiness without taking pain in their stride. Pain was the soul's experience of evolution...

The body had not yet been divorced from the soul, nor had sickness been divorced from pain. All words that indicated bodily pain were equally applicable to the suffering of the soul.

[The] raised threshold of physiologically mediated experience, which is characteristic of a medicalised society, makes it extremely difficult today to recognize in the capacity for suffering a possible symptom of health. The reminder that suffering is a responsible activity is almost unbearable to consumers, for whom pleasure and dependence on industrial outputs coincide.

During the 17th and 18th centuries, doctors who applied measurements to sick people were liable to be considered quacks by their colleagues. During the French Revolution, English doctors still looked askance at clinical thermometry, Together with the routine taking of the pulse, it became accepted clinical practice only around 1845, nearly thirty years after the stethoscope was first used by Laenne.

An advanced industrial society is sick-making because it disables people from coping with their environment and, when they break down, it substitutes a 'clinical' prosthesis for the broken *relationships.*

People would rebel against such an environment if medicine did not explain their biological disorientation as a defect in their health, rather than as a defect in the way of life which is imposed on them or which they impose on themselves.

The medical diagnosis of substantive disease entities that supposedly take shape in the individual's body is a surreptitious and amoral way of blaming the victim. The physician, himself a member of the dominating class, judges that the individual does not fit into an environment that has been engineered and is administered by other professionals, instead of accusing his colleagues of creating environments into which the human organism cannot fit.

Before sickness came to be perceived primarily as an organic or behavioural abnormality, he who got sick could still find in the eyes of the doctor a reflection of his own anguish and some recognition of the uniqueness of his suffering. Now, what he meets is the gaze of a biological accountant engaged in input/output calculations. His sickness is taken from him and turned into the raw material for an institutional enterprise. His condition is interpreted according to a set of abstract rules in a language he cannot understand. He is taught only about alien entities that the doctor combats, but only just as much as the doctor considers necessary to gain the patient's cooperation. Language is taken over by the doctors: the sick person is deprived of meaningful words for his anguish, which is thus further increased by linguistic mystification.

...while the industrial worker refers to his ache as a drab 'it' that hurts, his predecessors had many colourful and expressive names for the demons that bit or stung them.

Through the medicalisation of death, health care has become a monolithic world religion...

Like time-consuming acceleration, stupefying education, self-destructive military defence, disorienting information, or unsettling housing projects, pathogenic medicine is the result of industrial overproduction that paralyses autonomous action.

The patient is reduced to an object – his body – being repaired; he is no longer a subject being helped to heal. If he is allowed to participate in the repair process, he acts as the lowest apprentice in a hierarchy of repairmen. Often he is not even trusted to take a pill without the supervision of a nurse.

When people become aware of their dependence on the medical industry, they tend to be trapped in the belief that they are already hopelessly hooked. They fear a life of disease without a doctor much as they would feel immobilized without a car or bus.

Increasing and irreparable damage accompanies present industrial expansion in all sectors. In medicine this damage appears as iatrogenesis. Iatrogenesis is clinical when pain, sickness and death result from medical care; it is social when health policies reinforce an industrial organization that generates ill-health; it is cultural and symbolic when medically sponsored behaviour and delusions restrict the vital autonomy of people by undermining their competence in growing up, caring for each other, and aging, or when medical intervention cripples personal responses to pain, disability, impairment, anguish and death.

Man's consciously lived fragility, individuality, and relatedness make the experience of pain, of sickness, and of death an integral part of his life. The ability to cope with this trio autonomously is fundamental to his health. As he becomes dependent on the management of his intimacy, he renounces his autonomy and his health *must* decline. The true miracle of modern medicine is diabolical. It consists in making not only individuals but whole populations survive on inhumanly low levels of personal health. Medical nemesis is the negative feedback of a social organization that sets out to improve and equalize the opportunity for each man to cope in autonomy and ended by destroying it.

4. Biomedical Psychiatry – A Health Warning

Your symptoms – or those of your clients or patients if you are a counsellor or doctor – may themselves be effects of the very drugs that are being or have been prescribed to 'treat' them.

Recent decades have seen an enormous rise in the number of people treated with psychopharmaceutical medications – all of which have a direct effect on brain functioning. Such medications include:

Antidepressants (in particular so-called SSRI's which raise serotonin levels in the brain)

Anxiolytics (for treating anxiety, sleep problems and panic attacks – in particular the large range of so-called benzodiazepines such as Valium)

Neuroleptics (for treating so-called psychotic symptoms)

Stimulants (used on an increasing scale to treat children and adults with so-called behaviour disorders such as Attention Deficit Disorder)

Anticonvulsants (usually prescribed for epilepsy, fibromyalgia and neuralgias but some of which, for example pregabalin, are also prescribed for anxiety disorders)

What is not so well known is that many of the psychological and somatic symptoms treated by counsellors and psychotherapists, physicians and psychiatrists are a direct result of taking or having taken medications of these sorts.

Symptoms such as depression, anxiety, sleep disturbances, panic attacks, phobias, compulsions, mania, poor concentration, loss of affect, suicidal thoughts and psychotic episodes are all recognised by pharmaceutical companies themselves as potential effects of the very medications designed to treat them. Indeed it has been estimated that up to 50% of all patients attending mental health services may be presenting with anxiety disorders resulting from the use of anxiety-treating drugs or 'anxiolytics' – specifically the benzodiazepines. This is due to the development of dependency and acute or chronic withdrawal symptoms – such as increased anxiety or panic attacks – even whilst taking prescribed doses, whose efficacy declines as neuro-physiological habituation to the drugs or 'tolerance' sets in.

According to the psychiatrist Peter Breggin, health practitioners now confront a hidden epidemic of *iatrogenic* (medically caused) psychical and somatic illness resulting from short or long-term chemical disruption of brain functioning. The adverse effects of psychopharmaceutical medications, both acute and chronic, include:

- intended effects (for example the mind-numbing depression of brain functioning and the dulling of thought and emotion induced by *neuroleptics*).

- paradoxical effects (accentuation of the very symptoms which the drugs were prescribed to treat, such as panic attacks induced by *anxiolytics*).

- physiological side effects (ranging from respiratory, cardiac, gastrointestinal problems to long-term brain and liver damage, peripheral nerve damage, sexual dysfunction, weight gain, chronic fatigue or dyskinesia (uncontrolled Parkinsonian-type movements).

- psychological side effects (symptoms of mania, depression, panic attacks, psychotic episodes, suicidal ideation etc. of a sort not previously experienced by the individual at any time before taking the medications).

- withdrawal effects (acute or chronic psychological and physiological effects experienced when coming off prescribed medications).

- tolerance effects (needing ever-increasing dosages of the same drug to simply avoid what can be acute and frequent inter-dose withdrawal effects).

- short and long-term 'dependency' (in plain language addiction – resulting in tolerance and need for ever-higher doses to avoid withdrawal symptoms.)

There is a tendency to interpret even the most dangerous physiological side-effects – if reported – merely as symptoms of a patient's psychological disorder. Cardiac symptoms, for example, may be interpreted as 'anxiety' symptoms, rather than the other way round. As a result, patients with genuine cardiac problems may remain medically untested and untreated until they suffer a serious heart attack.

Many social workers, nurses and even GPs, counsellors, psychotherapists and alternative health practitioners however, still believe that the use and efficacy of psychopharmaceutical drugs is scientifically proven. The medical myth has it that mental disorders such as 'depression' are caused by biochemical imbalances in the brain. Not only has there never been any scientific evidence of this whatsoever, it is actually not technically possible to measure the levels of neurotransmitters in the synapses between brain cells. The hypothesis of an original 'chemical imbalance' was arrived at by arguing backwards from the supposedly therapeutic effects of drugs designed to chemically influence the release or reuptake of particular neurotransmitters – thereby altering their respective levels in the brain, even though the latter cannot be directly measured. Thus whilst there is no evidence that such drugs correct imbalances in the brain, they can be chemically guaranteed to cause them – artificially elevating or depressing neurotransmitter levels in a way that may affect not only mood, but all the body's most basic regulatory systems.

The principal 'evidence' for the therapeutic efficacy of psychopharmaceutical medications comes from short-term clinically controlled studies comparing the effects of an active drug with that of an inactive or 'inert' placebo. In most cases, the difference between the drug and placebo thought necessary to scientifically 'prove' the efficacy of the former is minimal. But comparing the effects of any active drug with an inert placebo is, as Peter Breggin says, misleading in itself. This is because the active drug may have its own type of placebo effect – giving the patient a felt sense of a drug's power by virtue of its felt effects, however subtle.

As John Grohol points out:

"...the double-blind placebo controlled study is not blind. Side effects are so obvious that more than 80% of the patients know whether they are on active medication or placebo, patients are equally accurate about other patients on the ward, and nurses and other personnel are privy as well. In some studies the only people who claim to be blind are the prescribing physicians, and in other studies the prescribing physicians admit being as aware of the patients' condition as everyone else." Even with active placebos *"the empirical data show that medication effect sizes are hard to distinguish from the placebo. Also not mentioned is that most antidepressant medications habituate, and the patients' symptoms return. Most patients believe they would feel even worse if they were not taking their medication."*

Grohol goes on to question the use of clinician-rated rather than patient-rated measures of 'improvement' in such trials, noting that:

"If patients cannot tell that they are better off in a controlled study, one must question the conventional wisdom about the efficacy of antidepressant drugs."

One of the main arguments in favour of the use of anti-depressants is suicide and violence prevention. How is it then, that several studies have shown an actual increase in suicide rates in those taking anti-depressants? How is that otherwise sober and responsible individuals with no history of violence or severe personality disorder can, within a few day or weeks fall victim to violent or suicidal impulses, even to the point of committing murder or suicide? One reason is the stimulant effect of the new Prozac-type antidepressants or Selective Serotonin Reuptake Inhibitors (SSRIs). The artificially elevated serotonin levels they are designed to induce can result not only in mild euphoria but manic states or psychotic syndromes similar to those produced by illegal amphetamines. Alternatively, they may, in the first few days of usage, result in an unnatural depression of serotonin levels as the brain tries to compensate for an artificially induced chemical imbalance. In both cases the drug has brought about a form of organic brain dysfunction of the very sort assumed, without evidence, to be responsible for the patient's symptoms. Another argument for the use of anti-depressants is their 'efficacy' for many people. No thought is given however, as to the reasons why such drugs are felt or deemed to be 'effective'. Breggin explains that:

"A patient typically is rendered unable to stay depressed during an episode of organic brain dysfunction, because depression requires a relatively intact brain and mind. Rendered either apathetic or artificially euphoric by brain dysfunction, the patient is evaluated as 'improved'."

"What psychiatrists call 'depression' – lethargy, apathy, nervousness, hopelessness, helplessness and unhappiness – is a serious problem often unrecognised as drug-related. Because of their depressant and debilitating effect, psychiatric drugs can make people feel so bad they want to kill themselves."

SSRI's such as *paroxetine* (Seroxat/Paxil) and Prozac may be authorised for use by patients over many years on the basis of clinical trials lasting from only 6 to 10 weeks. GlaxoSmithKline, whose sales of Seroxat/Paxil were valued at over one and a half billion pounds in 2000, continue aggressive marketing of the drug to doctors, with 100 million prescriptions given annually. This despite the fact that their own staff reported trial patients showing significant withdrawal symptoms of agitation and insomnia after only a short period on the drug – which now leads the World Health Organisation's list of pharmaceuticals reported by doctors to cause acute withdrawal problems. GSK leaflet accompanying prescriptions still tell the patient that "you cannot become addicted to Seroxat." No distinction is made between dependency of the sort comparable to an addict's cravings for tobacco or heroin, and addiction based purely on the need to avoid acute physical or psychological withdrawal symptoms.

The information leaflet for Seroxat also includes the following words:

"Occasionally, the symptoms of depression may include thoughts of harming yourself or committing suicide. Until the full antidepressant effect of your medication becomes apparent it is possible that these symptoms may increase in the first few weeks of treatment."

The tone is soothing. But in June 2001, GSK were forced to pay out $6.4 million in damages to the family of a man who killed his wife, daughter, granddaughter and then himself after only two days on Seroxat.

In contrast to the SSRIs, most *neuroleptic* drugs or 'anti-psychotics', together with the minor and major tranquillizers, work by dulling and depressing brain activity through a wide range of different neurotransmitters including dopamine and

GABA. The artificially-induced elevation or depression of mood brought on by the elevation or depression of different neurotransmitters in the brain, may have dramatic effects when the drug is *withdrawn* – either producing a dramatic 'rebound' elevation of neurotransmitter levels or leaving the brain incapable of generating normal neurotransmitter levels by itself. Breggin cites a typical example of withdrawal syndrome:

"Recently one of my patients, a young man in his twenties, was trying to taper off small doses of Elavil prescribed by another physician...within a day or two of complete withdrawal he began to feel ill. It seemed exactly like the flu. He felt lethargic and his muscles ached. He lacked appetite, felt sick to his stomach, and vomited in the morning.

Despite his tiredness he had trouble falling asleep and staying asleep. He felt increasing anxiety as well. A complete physical examination by an internist revealed no evidence of an infection, and I was forced to conclude that he had a typical flu-like withdrawal syndrome. He gradually recovered over a few weeks, vomiting for the last time about a month after ending the medication."

Not all are so 'lucky' as this patient. Countless harrowing stories by those who became unknowingly dependent on highly-addictive *benzodiazepine* tranquillizers and sleeping pills, or so-called 'non-addictive' anti-depressants, bear testament to the years or even decades of hell suffered in the attempt to withdraw from these drugs, and/or of the permanent post-withdrawal symptoms they still suffer.

With one out of four people in the UK thought to be suffering from a diagnosable mental disorder, the number of prescriptions of anti-depressants and anxiolytics is vast.

As long ago as 1984, it was reported by Professor Malcolm Lader that 11.2 percent of all adults took a *benzodiazepine* for anxiety or sleeping problems in any one year.

According to Lader:

'Even at a conservative estimate, 20% of these will develop symptoms when they attempt to withdraw. That means a quarter of a million people in the UK. It is now estimated that one and a half million people in the UK alone are chronically addicted to benzodiazepine anxiolytics such as diazepam (Valium) and lorazepam (Ativan). All the drugs in this class can induce dependency in a matter of days through suppressing the brain's natural production of anxiety- and stress-reducing neurotransmitters. Yet they account for 50% of global sales of psychopharmaceutical medications.'

Benzodiazepine use can also cause numerous *physical* health problems such as dental pains, abdominal disorders, acute neuralgias, muscle aches and a whole host of other symptoms – all of which may be misdiagnosed and mistreated by dentists, physicians and consultants unaware of this.

The whole situation was summed up by Vernon Coleman (*Life Without Tranquillizers*)

"The biggest drug-addiction problem in the world doesn't involve heroin, cocaine or marijuana. In fact, it doesn't involve an illegal drug at all. The world's biggest drug-addiction

problem is posed by a group of drugs, the benzodiazepines, which are widely prescribed by doctors and taken by countless millions of perfectly ordinary people around the world... Drug-addiction experts claim that getting people off the benzodiazepines is more difficult than getting addicts off heroin... For several years now pressure-groups have been fighting to help addicted individuals break free from their pharmacological chains. But the fight has been a forlorn one. As fast as one individual breaks free from one of the benzodiazepines another patient somewhere else becomes addicted. I believe that the main reason for this is that doctors are addicted to prescribing benzodiazepines just as much as patients are hooked on taking them."

The sheer scale of the problem with psychopharmaceutical medications becomes clear if we consider that probably 75% or more of so-called 'adverse reactions', including withdrawal symptoms and withdrawal syndromes, may be unreported. Worse still, they may be unrecognised as such by patients themselves, interpreted as signs of endogenous psychological disorders by physicians or psychotherapists, and/or treated by prescriptions of further psychiatric drugs. In an attempt to deal with recognised side-effects of these drugs, many psychiatrists and psychiatric health clinics around the world now regularly prescribe whole 'cocktails' of anti-depressant, neuroleptic and anxiolytic medications in the hope that they will chemically counter-balance each other's inherently toxic and unbalancing effects on brain functioning. At the same time pharmaceutical companies such as GSK are inventing ever new 'disorders' which can be 'treated' by drugs such as paroxetine. As well as 'panic disorder', 'obsessive compulsive disorder' the list now includes 'post-traumatic stress disorder' and 'social anxiety disorder' and 'attention deficit disorder'. Yet like standard DSM psychiatric designations such as 'bipolar disorder', 'personality disorder', these new 'disorder' terms seem to possess the authority of medical diagnoses – implying the existence of specific disease entities with an organic basis. In fact they are merely convenient labels for clusters of troublesome symptoms or behaviours that society has a problem understanding and responding to.

Biological psychiatry is founded on a flat denial that there is any meaning in 'mental illness', ignoring the simple fact that in a sick society or economy there may be good reasons for a person to feel anxious, depressed, disturbed, divided or driven to compulsive behaviours in order to cope. Illnesses in general are regarded as having biological 'causes' rather than meanings related to the individual's life.

Health itself is essentially defined only as the ability to 'function' normally as an employee – to cheerfully play one's part in sustaining a market economy in which all human relations are geared solely to commodity production and profit making. As a result, both medicine and psychiatry have both become tools of the 'therapeutic state' – their principal role being to manage or suppress all bodily or behavioural symptoms of the distress and dis-ease engendered by a sick society, not least with the help of drugs – thereby also turning them into a lucrative source of profit for the corporate health industry.

'Authoritarian psychiatry' is now being legitimised by governments all over the world through legislation, which denies mental patients the right to refuse medication and permits their enforced detention and drug 'treatment'. Given the enormous attention given by politicians and the media to the problems caused by illegal drugs and drug addiction, the failure by governments and health services to recognise the scale of addiction to legally prescribed drugs and the dangers of their adverse effects is hypocritical to say the least – amounting to a form of wilful ignorance. It is all the more important then, that social workers, mental health nurses, counsellors, psychotherapists and alternative health practitioners do not fall into the trap that so many orthodox physicians and psychiatrists have fallen into – that of accepting the medical and marketing myths perpetuated by pharmaceutical companies regarding the 'benefits' of psychiatric medications. Above all, it is important that they:

- obtain precise details of any client's present or past use, not only of illegal drugs but of legally prescribed medications, including the names of these medications and the length of time over which they were or have been taken.

- educate themselves in the adverse effects, addictive potentials and withdrawal symptoms of specific anxiolytic, anti-depressant and neuroleptic medications.

Thankfully, use of the internet now allows any patient or professional to quickly obtain information regarding specific drugs and drug types, as well as being host to many websites set up to support patients suffering from adverse reactions or dependency on such drugs, to inform health professionals of their dangers, to advise both patients and practitioners on safe methods of withdrawal, or simply to provide a forum in which users can share with each other the often horrifying experiences they have had of particular medications and their debilitating or life-destroying effects.

Recommended sites

www.benzo.org.uk - info on benzodiazepines
www.quitpaxil.org.uk - info on paroxetine (Paxil/Seroxat)
www.antidepressantfacts.com
www.Breggin.com - excellent articles by Peter Breggin
www.pssg.org - for Prozac survivors
www.antipsychiatry.org - the case against biopsychiatry
www.april.org.uk - on adverse drug reactions
www.mindfreedom.org - supporting patients
www.citawithdrawal.org.uk - Council for Information on Tranquillisers, Antidepressants and Painkillers

Recommended Reading

- Peter R. Breggin *Toxic Psychiatry*
- Breggin / Cohen *Your Drug May be Your Problem*
- Joan E.Gadsby *Addiction by Prescription*
- Heather Jones *Prisoner on Prescription*
- David Smail *The Nature of Unhappiness*
- Dr Ann Tracy *Prozac - Panacea or Pandora*

Further Reading and on-line Resources

Balint, Michael *The Doctor, the Illness and his Patient*

Boadella, David *Lifestreams*

Broom, Brian *Meaning-full Disease*

Chiozza, Luis A. *Hidden Affects in Somatic Disorders*

Chiozza, Luis A. *Why Do We Fall Ill? - The Story Hiding in the Body*

Foucault, Michel *The Birth of the Clinic*

Goldstein, Kurt *The Organism*

Heidegger, Martin *Zollikon Seminars*

Illich, Ivan *Limits to Medicine: Medical Nemesis - The Expropriation of Health*

Lakoff and Johnson, *Metaphors We Live By*

Lanctot, Guylaine *The Medical Mafia*

Leader, Darian and Cornfield, David *Why do People Get Ill?*

Lewontin, R. C. *Biology as Ideology*

Mindell, Arnold *Working with the Dreaming Body*

Roberts, Jane *The Way Toward Health - a Seth book*

Roberts, Janine *Fear of the Invisible*

Tauber, Alfred I. *The Immune Self*

Welch, Dr. H. Gilbert *Overdiagnosed: Making People Sick in the Pursuit of Health*

Wilberg, Peter *The Little Book of Hara* (Kindle e-book)

www.lifedoctoring.org.uk
www.existentialmedicine.org
www.heidegger.org.uk
www.thenewtherapy.org
www.thenewyoga.org

Other Books and Articles by Peter Wilberg

from PSYCHOSOMATICS to SOMA-SEMIOTICS - Felt Sense and the Sensed Body in Medicine and Psychotherapy New Yoga Publications 2010

Heidegger, Medicine and 'Scientific Method' New Gnosis Publications 2005

Meditation and Mental Health – an introduction to Awareness Based Cognitive Therapy New Yoga Publications 2010

The Therapist as Listener – Heidegger and the Missing Dimension of Counselling and Psychotherapy Training New Gnosis Publications 2005

The Awareness Principle – a Radical New Philosophy of Life, Science and Religion New Yoga Publications 2008

The QUALIA Revolution – from Quantum Physics to Qualia Science Second Edition, New Gnosis Publications 2008

Tantra Reborn – The Sensuality and Sexuality of our Immortal Soul Body New Yoga Publications 2009

The New Yoga of Awareness – Tantric Wisdom for Today's World New Yoga Publications 2209

The Science Delusion – Why God is Real and Science is Religious Myth New Gnosis Publications 2008

Event Horizon – Terror, Tantra and the Ultimate Metaphysics of Awareness New Yoga Publications 2008

Heidegger, Phenomenology and Indian Thought
New Gnosis Publications 2008

Deep Socialism – A New Manifesto of Marxist Ethics and Economics New Gnosis Publications 2003

From New Age to New Gnosis – Towards a New Gnostic Spirituality New Gnosis Publications 2003

Head, Heart and Hara – the Soul Centres of West and East New Gnosis Publications, 2003

Articles:

The Language of Listening
Journal of the Society for Existential Analysis 3

Introduction to Maieutic Listening
Journal of the Society for Existential Analysis 8.1

Listening as Bodywork
Energy and Character; Journal of Biosynthesis 30/2

The Language of Listening
Journal of the Society for Existential Analysis 3

From Existential Psychotherapy to Existential Medicine
Journal of the Society for Existential Analysis 22.2 July 2011

Index

Made in the USA
Lexington, KY
23 October 2013